PREVENTION OF CARDIOVASCULAR DISEASE

PREVENTION OF CARDIOVASCULAR DISEASE

Atherosclerosis,
Carotid Artery Disease,
Cerebral Artery Disease/Stroke,
Coronary Artery Disease,
Peripheral Artery Disease and
Hypertension

For Consumers, Healthcare Providers, Patients and Physicians

Eugene A. DeFelice, M.D.

iUniverse, Inc.
New York Lincoln Shanghai

Prevention of Cardiovascular Disease

Atherosclerosis, Carotid Artery Disease, Cerebral Artery Disease/Stroke, Coronary Artery Disease, Peripheral Artery Disease and Hypertension
For Consumers, Healthcare Providers, Patients and Physicians

iUniverse books may be ordered through booksellers or by contacting:

iUniverse
2021 Pine Lake Road, Suite 100
Lincoln, NE 68512
www.iuniverse.com
1-800-Authors (1-800-288-4677)

The author does not warrant, guarantee, or make any representation regarding use of any information contained in this book, or obtained from the Internet/Web as a result, in terms of being trustworthy, current, comprehensive, reliable, useful or otherwise. All information is provided "as is", and the reader assumes all risks that arise out of the use of this book and information contained therein, or from Web Resource(s)/Website(s) to which it may refer/pertain.

The reader should not substitute any information obtained via this book and/or the Internet/Web in any way for professional evaluation, advice, and/or diagnosis/ treatment by his/her own physician/healthcare provider.

ISBN-13: 978-0-595-36884-6 (pbk)
ISBN-13: 978-0-595-81297-4 (ebk)
ISBN-10: 0-595-36884-0 (pbk)
ISBN-10: 0-595-81297-X (ebk)

Printed in the United States of America

Dedication

This book is dedicated to Ms. Maryanne Harvey, M.S., who has devoted her professional career to the betterment of the health and welfare of others as a member of the New York State Department of Health, which she now serves as a consultant. Without Maryanne's able professional advice and assistance, publication of this book would not have been possible.

Contents

Preface

Most individuals do not live a healthy lifestyle or devote sufficient attention to their health and wellness. If you are one of those who do not, bear in mind that:

You may squander health in search of wealth
Work and toil and save
Then squander wealth in search of health
Only to find an early grave.

Anonymous

A healthy lifestyle is essential for good health and longevity. An unhealthy one often leads to chronic diseases such as cardiovascular disease (CVD), disability and a shortened lifespan. CVD refers to diseases of the heart and blood vessels which now accounts for over 30 percent of all worldwide deaths according to the World Health Organization. And, WHO estimates that by the year 2010, CVD is expected to become the leading cause of death worldwide.

Heart disease and stroke, the principal components of CVD, are now the first and third leading causes of death in the United States, accounting for more than 40 percent of all deaths. And around one million Americans die from CVD each year—CVD accounting for around 6 million hospitalizations each year in the US.

Most CVD in adults appears to be due largely to the "wrong way of life" and it is now estimated that over 50 percent of all CVD deaths/disability may be prevented by a combination of simple, cost-effective national efforts and individual initiatives and actions that reduce major modifiable risk factors for CVD such as an unhealthy lifestyle, high blood pressure, hyperlipidemia, overweight/obesity, smoking/secondhand smoke, sedentary lifestyle and stress.

While it is difficult to know the true cost of CVD, it is estimated to command a significant percentage of America's healthcare costs, perhaps as high as 3–5 percent. Vigorous, preventive measures are needed to help millions of Americans and others avoid unnecessary suffering due to CVD and bring down the now staggering costs to more reasonable levels.

Eugene A. DeFelice, MD

Acknowledgements

The author acknowledges that the Web health resources/websites in the Author' List in Chapter 10, and additional ones cited in the text as references, provided the information presented in this book and are hereby credited accordingly.

CHAPTER 1

▼

INTRODUCTION

1.1 DEFINITION OF CARDIOVASCULAR DISEASE

Cardiovascular disease (CVD) refers to diseases of the heart and blood vessels. "Cardio" refers to the heart and "vascular" to the entire arterial blood vessel system within the body including the brain, neck, chest, abdomen and legs.

1.2 WORLD HEALTH ORGANIZATION PROGRAM

The World Health Organization (WHO) program on CVD is concerned with the prevention, management, monitoring, and development of strategies to reduce the incidence, morbidity, and mortality of CVD by:
* effectively modifying/reducing risk factors and their determinants
* developing cost effective healthcare innovations for management

WHO now estimates that CVD:
* accounts for around 30 percent of total worldwide deaths
* 80 percent of CVD deaths now occur in low and middle income countries

- by the year 2010, CVD will become the leading cause of death in developing countries
- over 50 percent of all CVD deaths/disability may be prevented by a combination of simple, cost-effective national efforts, and individual initiatives and actions to reduce major risk factors such as high blood pressure (hypertension), hyperlipidemia (high blood cholesterol, etc.), overweight/obesity, smoking, and sedentary life style.

1.3 CARDIOVASCULAR DISEASE OVERVIEW

CVD is not a single disease but rather a group of heart and arterial blood vessel diseases. Heart disease and stroke, the principal components of CVD—are now the first and third leading causes of death in the United States accounting for more than 40 percent of all deaths. And, around one million Americans die of CVD each year, which amounts to one death every 33 seconds. Stroke alone accounts for disability in more than one million Americans. Although heart disease and stroke often are thought to affect men and older individuals primarily, CVD also is a major killer of women and people in the prime of life. It is estimated that almost 6 million hospitalizations each year are due to CVD.

Coronary artery disease (CAD), a leader among CVD, remains the leading cause of premature, permanent disability among working adults.

1.4 ECONOMIC IMPACT

The estimated economic impact of CVD on the U.S. healthcare system continues to grow larger as the population ages. In 2003, the cost of heart disease and stroke alone was estimated to be around $350 billion, $210 billion for healthcare expenditures and $140 billion for lost productivity from death and disability. While it is difficult to know the "true" cost, estimates now indicate that CVD involves a significant percentage of America's total healthcare costs. Measures are now needed to bring these costs down to more acceptable levels, and this most likely will occur largely through preventive measures.

1.5 Diseases Reviewed/Discussed

This book discusses the prevention of 6 of the major forms of CVD. These are: atherosclerosis, carotid artery disease, cerebral artery disease/stroke, coronary artery disease, peripheral artery disease and hypertension.

Additional information on CVD may be found at:
- National Center for Chronic Disease Prevention and Health Promotion
  Preventing Heart Disease and Stroke
  http://www.cdc.gov/nccdphp/bb_heartdisease/index.htm
- National Heart Lung and Blood Institute
  Heart and Vascular Diseases
  http://www.nhlbi.nih.gov/health/dci/Browse/Heart.html
- World Health Organization
  Cardiovascular Diseases
  http://www.who.int

1.6 Aspirin Prevention

A large number of clinical trials have shown that aspirin therapy provides a number of benefits in:

- people who have not yet developed symptoms or signs but are at sufficient risk for CVD
- almost all people who already have CVD

Aspirin is reported to prevent heart attack, stroke, and death in patients with known CVD. The United State Food and Drug Administration (FDA) has labeled aspirin as beneficial for patients with a previous heart attack, previous TIA and/or ischemic stroke, angina, and those who have undergone coronary bypass graft surgery or angioplasty.

Most healthcare providers recommend that patients with known CVD take up to 325 mg of aspirin daily. Higher doses apparently do not yield any greater benefit in terms of prevention of complications.

Aspirin can be life saving in patients who are actively having a heart attack. Healthcare providers recommend that most people suffering chest pain that is suspected of being a heart attack immediately take at least 325 mg of aspirin (a whole adult aspirin tablet) and seek medical attention immediately.

Aspirin also helps to prevent TIAs and stroke. Healthcare providers now recommend that most people who are at risk for a stroke or TIA begin taking 325 mg aspirin daily.

Large scale clinical trials have shown that aspirin prevents a first heart attack in people who have no signs or symptoms of cardiovascular disease (primary prevention).

However, the benefit for reducing the risk of a first heart attack must be weighed against potential adverse risks such as bleeding from the gastro-intestinal tract or in the brain. Thus various professional groups have concluded that aspirin should not be universally recommended for all healthy people to prevent a first heart attack or TIA or stroke but rather recommend daily aspirin for people in whom the CVD benefits outweigh the risks, which has been variably defined as those with a 10 year risk of developing heart disease of at least 6–10%, or those with a significant risk for a stroke.

Additional information on aspirin is available at:

- American Heart Association
  Aspirin in Heart Attack and Stroke Prevention
  http://www.americanheart.org/presenter.jhtml?identifier=4456

CHAPTER 2

▼

ATHEROSCLEROSIS

2.1 INTRODUCTION

Arteriosclerosis (hardening of the arteries) occurs when there is a thickening of the walls of the arteries in the body. This occurs with aging as a result of crosslinking of macromolecules in the arterial walls such as proteins and polysaccharides. As we age, some thickening of the walls of the arteries is believed to occur naturally.

The name, atherosclerosis, is derived from the Greek language and refers to the thickening of the arterial endothelium called sclerosis (hardening) due to accumulation of lipids (fat) and other substances called athere (gruel) that characterize the typical plaque lesion in the arteries. Such deposits/ plaques are associated with fibrosis, calcification and thickening of arteries. Unfortunately, today this process is almost always present, at least to some degree in most middle aged individuals, and especially in men over 45 and women over age 65 in the United States. And, atherosclerosis is now so prevalent that it is a leading cause of death in the US and the rest of the developed countries of the world.

Although many generalized or systemic risk factors are recognized to predispose individuals to the development of atherosclerosis, this disease preferentially affects certain key regions of the arterial circulation and corresponding organ systems including the brain, neck, heart and peripheral arterial system. In its severe forms, atherosclerosis leads to a more dramatic reduction in the size of the arterial lumen predisposing to ischemia (inadequate blood flow resulting in significant decrease in oxygenation of tissues), thrombosis and tissue/organ destruction.

The atherosclerotic process can lead to distinct clinical manifestations/disease, especially in its later stages, depending on the circulating bed/organ system affected and the characteristics of resulting lesions/pathology, which may be quite heterogenous.

2.2 RISK FACTOR CLASSIFICATION

Risk factors for atherosclerosis/CVD are basically divided into two categories, non-modifiable and modifiable.

Non-modifiable risk factors include such things as:

- age—CVD is more frequent with age, most becoming apparent after age 45–65
- family history—risk increases if present in parents, brothers, sisters, or children
- male gender—more prevalent in men compared to women
- menopause—women's risk increases after the menopause but does not quite reach male levels for age
- race—African Americans, Mexican Americans, Native Americans, and Asian Americans all have a higher risk

Modifiable risk factors also may be divided into two subcategories, namely major and contributing. Major risk factors are those that have been "proven" to significantly increase one's risk for CVD. Contributing risk factors, on the other hand, are regarded as those that may lead to an increased risk for CVD but their more exact role remains to be defined.

Patients/individuals need to know their modifiable risk factor profile and make necessary life style/other changes as early as possible in life, hopefully long before atherosclerotic disease becomes clearly manifest, in order to avoid complications and help achieve a healthier, happier, longer and more productive and enjoyable life.

Major modifiable risk factors and contributing modifiable risk factors are tabulated below for ease of reference.

Major Modifiable Risk Factors

- diabetes mellitus
- blood lipid abnormalities
- high blood pressure
- kidney disease
- metabolic syndrome x
- overweight/obesity
- periodontal disease
- physical inactivity
- psychological (emotional) stress
- smoking/secondhand smoke

Contributing Modifiable Risk Factors

- air pollution
- alcohol intake
- c-reactive protein
- hyperhomocysteinemia
- oral contraceptives
- oxidative stress/antioxidants

The more risk factors one has, the more likely it is for one to develop atherosclerosis and other forms of CVD. As indicated, some risk factors can be treated/modified for the better, and some cannot. By controlling as many risk factors as possible through lifestyle changes, diet, exercise, and prescription medicine, one can reduce risk and prevent atherosclerosis/CVD.

Additional information on risk factors is available at:
- American Heart Association
  Risk Factors for Coronary Heart Disease
  http://www.americanheart.org/presenter.jhtml?identifier=4726
- Cleveland Clinic Heart Center
  Preventing and Reversing Cardiovascular Disease
  http://www.clevelandclinic.org/heartcenter/pub/guide/prevention/riskfactors.htm
- Penn State Heart and Vascular Institute
  Risk Factors for Cardiovascular Disease
  http://www.hmc.psu.edu/heartandvascular/patient/articles/pe099.htm

- Texas Heart Institute
  Heart Disease Risk Factors
  http://www.texasheartinstitute.org/riskfact.html
- US Food and Drug Administration
  How to Keep Your Heart Healthy
  http://www.fda.gov/fdac/features/2003/603_heart.html
  Risk Factors for Cardiovascular Disease
  http://www.fda.gov/hearthealth/riskfactors/riskfactors.html

2.3 CLINICAL MANIFESTATIONS

Resulting clinical manifestations/disease from atherosclerosis include:
- carotid artery disease
- cerebral artery disease/stroke
- coronary artery disease
- peripheral artery disease
- hypertension

It now is estimated that around 35 percent of the adult population, or over 60 million persons, live with some form of atherosclerosis/CVD. And, the percentage affected is much higher in those over age 65.

2.4 PREVENTION

The primary prevention of atherosclerosis and its complications (other CVD) is the goal and presents a long term challenge to all healthcare professionals and individuals alike.

Physicians, healthcare workers and organizations especially need to counsel patients regarding the need for CVD risk factor modification including:

- the health risks of smoking/secondhand smoke, and provide guidance concerning smoking cessation
- control of alcohol intake, diabetes, high blood pressure, and stress (both psychological and oxidative)
- prudent dietary/nutritional considerations
- proper exercise program
- need to achieve and maintain normal weight

2.5 UCLA ATHEROSCLEROSIS PROGRAM

Atherosclerosis is a progressive disease. While the short-term prognosis may be improved with medical management and revascularization strategies, the underlying atherosclerotic disease process must be addressed in order to improve long-term patient outcome. One of the best ways to do this is illustrated by the UCLA School of Medicine's Comprehensive Atherosclerosis Treatment Program.

The UCLA program is based on a great deal of clinical/scientific evidence demonstrating that treatment alters the natural history of the disease, improves clinical outcomes, and prolongs survival. The goal, whether it be during hospitalization or an outpatient visit for any reason, in a patient with CVD is to ensure the initiation and maintenance of clinical trial evidence—based therapies. Patients with diabetes have similar cardiovascular risk as patients with established atherosclerosis and should also be targeted for treatment, irrespective of symptoms, presence of atherosclerosis, or degree of glycemic control.

UCLA takes the position that therapies that have been demonstrated to lower the risk of subsequent morbidity/mortality in patients with atherosclerosis include aspirin, cholesterol lowering medications, angiotensin converting enzyme inhibitors (ACE), omega-3 fatty acids, exercise, and smoking cessation. Beta blockers lower the risk of myocardial infarction in patients with coronary artery disease, other atherosclerotic vascular disease or diabetes, as well as prolong survival in patients with acute coronary syndromes (ACS) and those with heart failure. Despite the clinical evidence supporting their use, these survival enhancing therapies are underutilized when guided by conventional care. Accordingly, the UCLA treatment program guidelines are reported to aim at optimizing the initiation and maintenance of the definitive evidence-based treatments for atherosclerosis including the following:

- diagnostic and therapeutic focus for patients with carotid artery disease, coronary artery, cerebral artery or other vascular disease, and diabetes should shift to address the underlying atherosclerosis

- patients with coronary artery, other arterial disease, and/or diabetes should be treated with therapies that have been demonstrated in randomized clinical trials to alter the natural history of atherosclerosis, decrease cardiovascular adverse events, and improve survival

- patients should be treated regardless of whether they have undergone or are undergoing a revascularization procedure and regardless of whether they have symptomatic angina, silent ischemia, or atherosclerosis without ischemia

- antiplatelet agent, beta blocker, ACE inhibitor, statin, omega-3 fatty acids, diet, and an aerobic exercise program should be considered initial and fundamental therapy for all patients with clinical manifestations of any atherosclerotic arterial disease (coronary artery disease, cerebral artery disease, peripheral artery disease, or carotid artery disease) and/or diabetes irrespective of the presence or absence of known vascular disease.

- patients with documented atherosclerosis or diabetes should not be discharged from the hospital or leave their outpatient encounter without initiation of treatment, unless contraindicated. Such treatment is reported to consists of:
  - aspirin—started and continued in all patients.
  - alternatively, clopidrogel—started in aspirin allergic or intolerant patients. The combination of aspirin plus clopidrogel is recommended in the acute coronary syndrome, post stent, and other high-risk patients.
  - statin therapy—started in all atherosclerotic arterial disease patients and/or patients with diabetes irrespective of baseline LDL cholesterol. Lipid levels to be targeted in patients with coronary artery, other arterial diseases, or diabetes include: LDL <70 mg/dl, HDL > 40 mg/dl, TG < 150 mg/Dl.
  - ACE inhibitors—to be started in all patients even if the blood pressure and ejection fraction are normal, irrespective of renal function
  - angiotension receptor antagonists (ARA)—to be provided if ACE inhibitor therapy is not tolerated or has unacceptable side effects
  - beta blockers—to be started in all patients, including those with heart failure and diabetes
  - aldosterone antagonists—to be considered in patients who are post myocardial infarction with a left ventricular ejection frac-

    tion of 40 or less, with signs or symptoms of heart failure or diabetes have reduced mortality on aldosterone antagonists.

- omega-3 fatty acids—to be started in all patients and patients should be provided with dietary instructions, including ideal weight/body mass index

- an aerobic exercise program to be prescribed—consisting of moderate intensity activity 30–60 minutes, a minimum of 5 days per week
- patients to be strongly encouraged to stop smoking and formal cessation Rx/referral provided.

Therapies such as nitrates and calcium channel blockers that provide symptomatic benefit but have not been shown to decrease mortality or the incidence of coronary events to be reserved for patients who remain unacceptably symptomatic despite aforementioned recommended therapies.

Patients with established carotid artery, cerebral artery, coronary artery and peripheral arterial atherosclerosis are at high risk for adverse vascular events and death regardless of identifiable risk factors and regardless of whether they have undergone revascularizaton. However, combination cardiovascular protective therapy targeting the underlying atherosclerotic disease process, and risk factor modification can markedly improve clinical outcome in patients whereas failure to employ these therapies increases patient morbidity/mortality. Compliance and treatment utilization is reported to be enhanced by employing secondary prevention measures prior to hospital discharge. The UCLA treatment program recommends that patients not be discharged from the hospital without initiation of definitive atherosclerosis treatment, unless contraindications exist and are documented.

2.6 TREATMENT GOALS

In addition to aforementioned therapies, the UCLA program recommends that the following treatment goals should be achieved in a timely fashion and maintained, with careful documentation in the patient medical record, namely:

- LDL < 70 mg/dl—once achieved, document biannual or annual lipid panel
- BP < 140/90 mmHg—document on each follow-up visit, with additional monitoring as indicated
- BP < 130/80 mmHg—if diabetic or in renal failure.
- not smoking—current status with regards to smoking should be documented in all current/former smokers. Recommendations for smoking cessation and nicotine replacement and behavior modification attempts should be documented.
- HbA1C < 7.0%—diabetes management/tight control
- aerobic physical activity program 30–60 minutes/day, 5–7 days a week

The UCLA School of Medicine Cardiovascular Hospitalization Atherosclerosis Management Program: CHAMP treatment algorithm and further details regarding the program are available at: http://www.ucla.edu/champ/action.htm

Additional information on atherosclerosis is available at:
- National Heart Lung and Blood Institute
  What is Atherosclerosis
  http://www.nhlbi.nih.gov/health/dci/Diseases/Atherosclerosis/Atherosclerosis_WhatIs.html

CHAPTER 3

▼

CAROTID ARTERY DISEASE

3.1 INTRODUCTION

Carotid Artery Disease results from atherosclerosis of the carotid arteries and their branches. The two external carotid arteries, one on each side of the neck, supply blood to the brain and eyes. The beginning of the internal carotid artery and the middle or anterior cerebral artery are the most common sites of atherosclerosis. A superimposed clot leads to a TIA (transient ischemic attack) or a stroke. Intracranial atherosclerotic sites predominate in African Americans and Asians. Rarely, the beginning of the common carotid artery may be the site of the initial atherosclerotic lesion.

Emboli into the internal carotid artery may cause temporary occlusion of the ophthalmic artery branches causing monocular blindness (known as amaurosis fugax). This event sometimes appears like a curtain descending over all or part of one's vision in the affected eye and may last for only a short while or for several hours.

3.2 RISK FACTORS

Risk factors for carotid artery disease include all those for atherosclerosis listed previously in section 2.2. Those of particular interest for carotid artery disease are:

- family history of atherosclerosis (coronary artery disease, stroke, cerebral artery disease or peripheral artery disease)
- age (greater in men than women less than age 75 but higher in women after age 75)
- TIA (transient ischemic attack)
- atherosclerosis of blood vessels of eye discovered during routine eye exam
- carotid artery bruit discovered during routine physical exam
- smoking/secondhand smoke
- diabetes mellitus
- overweight/obesity
- high blood LDL (low density lipoprotein cholesterol)—although this risk is not as strong as it is for coronary artery disease
- hypertension
- sedentary lifestyle

If one already has coronary artery disease, one is more likely to develop carotid artery disease.

A temporary blockage of the blood supply to the brain (TIA) may be the first sign of carotid artery disease. Muscle weakness on one side of the face or numbness of an arm or leg which usually lasts for about an hour or up to 24 hours may occur.

One of the first signs of blockage of the blood supply to the brain and eyes may be revealed on routine examination of the blood vessels of the eye(s). Evidence of atherosclerosis of the retinal arterial blood vessels may be the first indication of impending blockage of the internal carotid artery, or the ophthalmic artery (the first branch off the internal carotid), or its branch (the central retinal artery).

Another early sign of carotid artery disease is a carotid bruit heard over the external carotid arteries in the neck in a routine physical exam. A carotid bruit is an abnormal "rushing" sound largely due to blood turbulence over plaque formation heard when using a stethoscope to listen to blood flow in the carotid arteries. One may even hear the carotid bruit in one's own ear.

A carotid bruit indicates a fatty buildup and stenosis (atherosclerosis) in the carotid artery. However, a carotid bruit doesn't necessarily mean that the stenosis will worsen and a TIA/stroke will result. Nevertheless, a carotid bruit does usually indicate carotid artery disease and a higher risk for TIA and or stroke until proven otherwise.

Thus, a carotid bruit, TIA, or amaurosis fugax are significant risk factors and early warning signs that a serious problem involving the brain's blood supply and carotid artery disease may exist. And, each of these early warning signs usually can be easily ascertained via careful patient history and routine physical examination.

3.3 DIAGNOSIS

During a history and physical exam, a physician will inquire about symptoms and signs of a TIA or stroke such as muscle weakness, speech or vision difficulties, or lightheadedness. Using a stethoscope, a physician may hear the rushing sound (bruit) in the affected carotid artery. Unfortunately even dangerous levels of carotid artery disease sometimes fail to produce such a sound. And, even some lesser carotid stenosis (blockages) with low risk may result in a bruit.

In most cases, after a history and physical exam and lab tests, further testing/evaluation is usually needed to establish the diagnosis of carotid artery disease. These may include:

- ultrasound imaging
- arteriography
- magnetic resonance angiography (MRA)

Frequently these procedures are carried out in a stepwise fashion: from a physician's evaluation of history, physical exam, and assessment of signs and symptoms—to ultrasound—to arteriography—to MRA for increasingly difficult cases.

Ultrasound imaging is a painless, noninvasive procedure in which sound waves, above the range of human hearing are sent into the neck in the area of the carotid arteries. Echoes bounce off the moving blood and tissue in the carotid artery and form an image which shows either no disease, or varying degrees of blockage and impaired blood flow. Ultrasound is fast, risk free, relatively inexpensive and painless compared to arteriography and MRA.

Arteriography is used to confirm findings of ultrasound imaging which can lead to uncertain findings in some cases. Arteriography employs x-rays of the carotid artery taken when a special contrast dye is injected into the carotid artery. An arteriogram is more specific and expensive to do and carries its own small risk of complications including a stroke.

Magnetic Resonance Angiography (MRA) is a relatively new imaging technique that avoids most of the risks associated with arteriography. An MRA uses magnetism instead of x-rays to create the image of the carotid arteries—thus it is considered to be safer—however it is the most expensive of the three procedures.

3.4 PREVENTION

Primary prevention of carotid artery disease involves the management of modifiable risk factors for atherosclerosis. If one:

- smokes, stop—avoid secondhand smoke
- has hypertension—take measures to normalize your blood pressure,
- is sedentary—engage in physical activities and exercise
- manifests abnormal blood lipid levels—modify levels to acceptable limits with diet, exercise and medication
- is diabetic—establish measures to ensure tight control of blood glucose and lipid levels
- feels stressed—reduce or minimize stress levels and learn to cope effectively

3.5 SURGICAL TREATMENT

Most individuals with carotid artery disease don't need surgery and can be managed medically. While the vast majority of persons over age 75 have some degree of carotid artery disease, they usually are asymptomatic and the disease process may be of little concern. However, one should begin to become concerned when carotid artery plaques grow and stenosis (blockage) proceeds beyond the 50 percent level. Once 70 percent blockage occurs, or if the carotid artery disease causes symptoms/signs like a TIA or amaurosis fugax, then one is usually considered to have severe carotid artery disease.

Individuals with severe stenosis in their carotid arteries should be considered for surgical treatment in a procedure called an endarterectomy. Numerous large clinical studies in the United States and Europe have confirmed that carotid endarterectomy for advanced carotid artery disease is superior in preventing stroke compared with the best medical treatment available. In fact, patients receiving medical treatment alone are at least 2–3 times more likely to have a stroke compared with those surgically treated with an endarterectomy.

Endarterectomy removes plaque from inside the carotid artery wall and restores adequate blood flow to the brain. This surgical procedure may be employed successfully because plaque blockage/stenosis generally is limited to a small defined area of the carotid artery in the neck. This allows surgery to be done through a small incision in the neck and carotid artery to remove the obstructing plaque. In most cases, the surgical procedure goes well and the patient can go home the morning or so after surgery.

Carotid endarterectomy surgery has been found to be highly beneficial even for persons who already have had a stroke, or experienced warning signs of a stroke and have a severe stenosis of 70–99%. In this group surgery reduces the estimated 2 year risk of stroke by more than 80 percent from greater than 1 in 4 to less than 1 in 10. This surgery reduces the 5 year risk of stroke by only 6.5 percent for patients with a 50–69% stenosis compared to an 80 percent risk reduction for patients with 70 percent or greater stenosis. Patients with 50 percent stenosis or lower usually do not derive enough benefit from endarterectomy to outweigh the risks of the procedure.

Surgery carries a certain risk in that it may result in a stroke or other complications. Important risk factors for a post surgical stroke include the degree of stenosis, gender, symptoms/signs, and degree of blockage/stenosis of the carotid artery on the opposite side. Without complicating illnesses, age alone is not an important risk. However, combinations of risk factors can greatly increase a person's chances of having a stroke from the surgical procedure and can increase the likelihood of other complications as well.

Early results with carotid artery angioplasty and stent placement to relieve blockage/stenosis in the carotid arteries also are beginning to show promise in the treatment of carotid artery disease.

Additional information on surgical treatment of carotid artery disease is available at:
- Cleveland Clinic Heart Center
  Carotid Artery Disease
  http://www.clevelandclinic.org/heartcenter/pub/guide/disease/vascular/carotidartery.htm

- Medlineplus
  Carotid Artery Disease
  http://www.nlm.nih.gov/medLinplus/carotidarterydisese.html
- National Institute of Neurological Disorders and Stroke
  Questions and Answers about Carotid Endarterectomy
  http://www.ninds.nih.gv/disorders/stroke/carotid_endarterectomy_
  backgrounder.htm

CHAPTER 4

CEREBRAL ARTERY DISEASE/STROKE

4.1 INTRODUCTION

Strokes rank as the third leading "killer disease" in the United States. Each year more than 700,000 Americans have a stroke and up to 200,000 die from stroke-related causes. The incidence of stroke increases with age and affects many people in their "golden years".

A stroke occurs when the blood supply to a part of the brain fails and brain cells die due to the resulting lack of oxygen. Although some brain cell injury is reversible, death of brain cells is permanent, usually leaving lasting disability. Strokes occur in all age groups, in both sexes, and in all races/ethnic groups in every country. A stroke is more common and deadly in African-Americans.

4.2 CLASSIFICATION OF STROKE

There are two broad categories of stroke, namely those:
- caused by a blockage of blood flow (ischemic)
- due to bleeding/hemorrhage (hemorrhagic)

While not usually fatal, a blockage of a blood vessel in the brain or neck is called an ischemic stroke, and is the most frequent cause of stroke being responsible for up to 90% of the cases. Such blockages stem from three basic conditions, namely:

- formation of a clot within a blood vessel of the brain (i.e. internal carotid artery) or neck (external carotid artery), called thrombosis
- the movement of a clot from another part of the body such as the heart to the neck or brain, called an embolism
- severe narrowing of an artery in, or leading to, the brain called athero-sclerotic stenosis

Bleeding into the brain or spaces surrounding the brain produces the second type of stroke, called hemorrhagic stroke, an often fatal condition.

4.3 WARNING SIGNS OF STROKE

Warning signs of a stroke are clues the body provides indicating that the brain may not be receiving enough blood/oxygen. Such signs may include the sudden occurrence of:

- numbness or weakness of the face, arm, or leg, especially on one side
- confusion, trouble speaking, or understanding
- trouble seeing in one or both eyes
- difficulty walking, dizziness, loss of balance or coordination
- severe headache with no known cause

Sometimes warning signs may last only a little while and then disappear completely. These brief episodes, known as TIAs (transient ischemic attacks), are often referred to as "mini strokes".

Usually a TIA is manifested by a neurological deficit generally lasting less than 24 hours (typically 5 to 20 minutes). The neurological deficit is generally focal and confined to an area of the brain perfused by a specific artery. Although brief, a TIA identifies an underlying serious arterial condition that signifies an immediate need for medical help.

4.4 Risk Factors for TIA/Stroke

Risk factors for a TIA/stroke are essentially the same as for atherosclerosis and are outlined in section 2.2

A risk factor is a condition or behavior that occurs more frequently in those who are at greater risk of having a TIA/stroke. Having a risk factor for a TIA/stroke doesn't mean that one will have a stroke, and not having a risk factor doesn't mean one will avoid a TIA/stroke. However, it is clear that the risk of a TIA/stroke increases with the number and severity of risk factors present.

4.5 Prevention/Treatment

Modifiable risk factors for the prevention of a TIA/stroke include:

Medical conditions

- carotid artery disease
- cigarette smoking
- coronary artery disease
- diabetes mellitus
- elevated blood homocysteine
- elevated C-reactive protein
- hyperlipidemia
- hypertension
- metabolic syndrome x
- overweight/obesity
- TIA

Behaviors

cocaine abuse
dietary factors
excessive alcohol intake
physical inactivity
psychological stress
smoking/secondhand smoke
unhealthy lifestyle

Hypertension (high blood pressure) is by far one of the most potent risk factors for a TIA/stroke. Blood pressure needs to be checked periodically and if high, a strategy needs to be worked out to bring it down to normal levels (<140/90 and preferably down to <120/80) to increase chances for prevention.

Carotid artery disease also remains one of the stronger risk factors for a TIA or stroke, especially when the stenosis (blockage) is greater than 50 percent. The carotid arteries are the main blood vessels in the neck supplying blood/oxygen to the brain and blockage of one or more of these arteries is one of the leading causes of stroke in Americans. Thus, when discovered, consideration needs to be given to ways to reduce stenosis including surgical intervention (endarterectomy).

Cigarette smoking also is a major risk factor linked to TIA and stroke. Approximately 20 percent of strokes are attributable to cigarette smoking. Nicotine in tobacco smoke is known to raise blood pressure. Carbon monoxide in smoke reduces the amount of oxygen blood can carry to the brain. And, smoking is known to "thicken" the blood making it more likely to clot and produce a TIA/stroke. By quitting smoking at any age, the risk of TIA or stroke is reduced significantly. Programs and medications are now available to help stop smoking. The Framingham study found that stroke risk returns to the same level as non smokers around five years after cessation.

The American Heart Association recommends immediate smoking cessation advice/counseling be given to all current smokers who have experienced a TIA or stroke.

Heart disease, valve defects, irregular heart beat, and enlargement of the heart's chambers can result in blood clots that may break loose (embolus) and lodge in a blood vessel leading to the brain and result in a TIA or stroke. Aspirin and anticoagulant and antiarrhythmic agents may help prevent such episodes from occurring.

Diabetes not only affects the body's ability to utilize glucose but it also produces destructive atherosclerotic changes in the endothelium of arterial blood vessels throughout the body, including the blood supply to the brain. In patients with diabetes and metabolic syndrome x, a TIA or stroke may occur more frequently and be correspondingly more severe. Proper management of diabetes and metabolic syndrome x can decrease the risk of a TIA/stroke accordingly.

A TIA should receive emergency medical attention since it may be signaling the subsequent occurrence of a "full blown" ischemic stroke. Aspirin is considered to be very useful in preventing TIAs and strokes and their reoccurrence.

Statin drugs are reported to be independently protective against recurrent TIAs and stroke whereas no protective effect has been found for warfarin or antiplatelet drugs. Simvastatin is reported to reduce not only the risk of a heart attack but also a TIA or stroke. In the ASCOT—LLA (Anglo-Scandinavian Cardiac Outcomes Trial) clinical trial, atorvastatin also was associated with a highly significant reduction of stroke.

Physical inactivity remains an important independent risk factor for stroke. And exercise has established its benefits in stroke prevention. Exercise may confer stroke prevention through a variety of ways including:
- improvement in hypertension and diabetes control
- increase in plasma tissue plasminogen activator reducing occurrence of thrombosis
- increase in HDL, reduction in LDL blood cholesterol
- decrease in fibrinogen levels
- decrease in platelet stickiness

The Center for Disease Control and Prevention as well as the National Institutes of Health and the Institute of Medicine recommend that every American adult should exercise for at 30–60 (preferably 60) minutes daily 5–7 (preferably 7) days a week. Benefits of exercise are apparent even for moderate activities such as brisk walking.

Numerous studies have confirmed the inverse association between fruit and vegetable intake and stroke. Studies have shown that an increment of 1 serving of fruits and vegetables is associated with a 6 percent lower risk of ischemic stroke. Daily intake of fruits and vegetables provides a 25–35% reduction in ischemic stroke mortality.

Low potassium intake and low serum potassium are associated with increased stroke mortality. Diuretic users are reported to have increased risk for stroke associated with lower serum potassium. Potassium and magnesium supplementation and diets high in fiber may reduce a person's risk of stroke by as much as 38 percent according to recent evidence.

The Nurses' Health Study demonstrated a significant reduction in the risk of ischemic/thrombotic stroke in individuals consuming fish 2 times per week. No beneficial association was observed between consumption of fish or fish oil and hemorrhagic stroke. The Health Professional Follow-Up Study found that men who consumed fish 1–3 times a month had significantly less episodes of stroke than those who consumed fish less than once a month.

Moderate alcohol consumption is reported to lower the risk of stroke. However, high or excessive alcohol intake is associated with up to 10 fold increased risk of stroke. Moderate alcohol intake is limited to 1–2 small alcohol drinks per day for men and 1 drink per day for women.

A calorie restricted diet low in saturated fat and cholesterol, low in sodium, high in potassium and calcium, and containing 5–9 (preferably 9) servings of fruits and vegetables plus whole grains and 2 servings per week of fatty fish such as salmon or tuna, may reduce high blood pressure as much as antihypertensive drugs, and may be more effective than statin drugs in reducing death from stroke and myocardial infarction. Such a diet, rich in natural proportions of vitamins and minerals as well as antioxidants, may also provide some benefits that we are only beginning to define and understand.

Addition information on stroke/prevention is available at:

- American Academy of Family Practice
  Stroke: Warning Signs and Tips for Prevention
  http://www.familydoctor.org/290.xml
  Stroke: Part II, Management of Acute Ischemic Stroke
  http://www.aafp.org/afp/990515ap/2828.html
- American Heart Association
  Prevention of Heart Disease and Stroke
  http://www.americanheart.org.presenter.jhtml?identifier=3010152
- National Institute Neurological Disorders and Stroke
  What You Need to Know About Stroke
  http://www.ninds.nih.gov/disorders/stroke/stroke_needtoknow.htm
- UCLA School of Medicine
  Protect: Preventing Reoccurrence of Thromboembolic Events through Coordinated Treatment
  http://strokeprotect.mednet.ucla.edu

CHAPTER 5

▼

CORONARY ARTERY DISEASE

5.1 INTRODUCTION

Coronary artery disease (CAD) may be referred to under different names such as coronary heart disease (CHD), heart disease (HD), and ischemic heart disease (IHD). For the purposes of this book, it will be referred to as CAD.

Over 13–15 million individuals in the United States have CAD. Coronary artery disease now is the most common, serious, chronic, life-threatening illness in the US and causes more deaths, disability and economic costs than any other CVD. Each year more than half a million Americans die from CAD and it remains the number one killer of both men and women.

Coronary arteries are a major site for atherosclerotic disease. Postmortem studies on accident victims and military casualties have demonstrated that coronary atherosclerosis probably begins prior to age 20 in many cases, and even in infancy in some individuals. It becomes widespread among adults after ages 45–65, even in those who remain asymptomatic during life. Asymptomatic individuals without any history or manifestations of coronary artery disease often show microscopic scars secondary to myocardial infarction in regions supplied by diseased vessels.

The major epicardial coronary arteries are the main sites of atherosclerosis. CAD occurs when the arteries that supply blood to the heart muscle become hardened and narrowed due to buildup of plaque on the inner walls or lining of the arteries. Blood flow to the heart is reduced as plaque narrows the coronary arteries and decreases the oxygen supply to the heart muscle. The major risk factors for atherosclerosis are thought to disturb the normal function of the coronary vascular endothelium in these coronary artery beds leading to CAD.

Studies have shown that when a stenosis caused by atherosclerosis disease reduces the coronary artery lumen by approximately 70–75 percent, a full range of increases in blood flow needed to meet increased heart demand is no longer possible. And, when the coronary lumen is reduced by 80 percent or more blood flow at rest may be so reduced/compromised that any further minor decreases can result in more dramatic falls in blood flow causing ischemia, angina and myocardial infarction.

5.2 PATHOPHYSIOLOGY

In CAD, plaque deposits made up of fat, cholesterol, calcium, and other substances from blood buildup in the coronary arteries. While plaque buildup often begins in childhood, over time it can:
- narrow the arteries so that less blood can flow to the heart muscle
- completely block the arteries and flow of blood
- cause blood clots to form and block the arteries.

Plaque in the coronary arties can be:

- hard and stable. Hard plaque causes the artery walls to thicken and harden. This condition is associated more with angina than with a heart attack.

- soft and unstable. Soft plaque is more likely to break open/apart and cause a blood clot (thrombosis). This usually leads to a heart attack (myocardial infarction).

Overtime, CAD can weaken the heart muscle involved and contribute to:

- heart failure—a condition in which the heart is not able to pump sufficient blood to the rest of the body effectively. Heart failure does not mean that the heart has stopped or is about to stop working. However, it does mean that the heart is failing to pump necessary blood/oxygen the way it should for the rest of the body to function normally.

- arrhythmias—are changes in the normal rhythm of the heartbeats. These can be quite serious and life threatening if not controlled by proper therapy.

5.3 Risk Factors

Major risk factors for coronary artery disease are essentially the same as those listed for atherosclerosis. In order to prevent coronary artery disease, risk factors for atherosclerosis need to be assessed and optimized in any given individual patient as early as possible in the disease process.

Risk factors are conditions that make it more likely that one will develop CAD. Those factors that you cannot do anything about are:

- age—risk for CAD increases in men after age 45, and in women, after age 55
- family history of premature heart disease—diagnosed before age 55 in father or brother or before age 65 in mother or sister.
- gender—CAD is more common in males

Risk factors that one can do most about include:
- alcohol consumption
- diabetes mellitus
- diet/nutrition
- high blood pressure
- high LDL cholesterol/triglycerides
- kidney disease
- metabolic syndrome x
- overweight/obesity
- physical inactivity
- psychological stress

The more risk factors present in any given individual, the greater the probability for developing CAD. Chapter 8 provides further information on modifiable risk factors for CVD.

5.4 Symptoms/Signs

The most common symptoms of CAD are:
- chest pain/discomfort (angina), or pain in one or both arms, the left shoulder, neck, jaw or back
- shortness of breath
- fatigues easily

Most cases of myocardial ischemia are characterized by chest discomfort/ pain due either to angina pectoris and/or myocardial infarction. Having entered into a symptomatic phase, an individual may exhibit a stable or progressive course, revert to the asymptomatic stage of the disease process, or suddenly die.

Severity of symptoms varies widely and they may become more severe as the coronary arteries become narrower due to buildup of plaque in the atherosclerotic process. In some people, the first sign of CAD is a heart attack (myocardial infarction). This usually occurs when plaque in a coronary artery leads to a blood clot—in up to 50 percent of cases. In others, a clot is not involved but things such as coronary artery spasm may be.

Myocardial infarction is one of the most common diagnoses in hospitalized patients in industrialized countries including the United States where over 2 million cases occur annually.

The mortality rate from myocardial infarction in the US is around 30 percent with about half these deaths occurring before the patient reaches the hospital. Although the mortality rate after hospital admission for myocardial infarction has declined by about 30 percent over the last 2 decades, approximately 2–4% of patients surviving the initial stay in the hospital, die in the first year after a myocardial infarction. Survival is further reduced in those over 65 where the mortality rate is around 20 percent at one month and about 35 percent at one year.

In approximately one half of cases of myocardial infarction, a key precipitating factor is present such as vigorous exercise, severe emotional stress, or a medical illness or surgery.

5.5 Diagnosis

There is no single test to diagnose CAD. History, physical exam, a battery of lab tests, and risk factor and symptom assessments are used to decide which of the following tests/procedures to perform:

- EKG (electrocardiogram}—to measure the rate and regularity of heart beat
- echocardiogram—to create a picture of the heart and assess various aspects of cardiac function using sound waves
- exercise stress test—to show how well the heart pumps blood at higher work levels when it needs more oxygen. EKG and BP readings usually are taken before, during and after exercise to see how the heart responds to exercise. The first EKG and blood pressure readings are done to obtain a baseline. Readings then are taken while walking on an exercise treadmill, or pedaling a stationary bicycle, or receiving medicine to make the heart beat faster. The test continues until a target heart rate is reached that has been set by the physician doing the test. The exercise part is stopped if an EKG rhythm abnormality, chest pain/discomfort, or a very sharp rise in blood pressure occurs. Monitoring continues for 10 to 15 minutes after exercise or until heart rate returns to baseline.
- chest x-ray—to take a picture of the heat and lungs looking for any cardiac and/or pulmonary pathology
- cardiac catherization—to examine the inside of the arteries to determine the degree any blockage (stenosis). This test involves passing a

thin flexible tube through the femoral artery in the groin (top of the leg) or in the arm to reach the coronary arteries. With this procedure, the doctor can determine pressure and blood flow in the heart chambers, collect blood samples, and examine the arteries of the heart using x-ray

- coronary angiography—to visualize the flow of blood through the heart on an x-ray screen. This usually is performed along with cardiac catherization using a dye, for contrast, injected into the coronary arteries

- nuclear heart scan—to outline heart chambers and major blood vessels leading to and from the heart to reveal any damage to heart muscle using radioactive tracers (technetium or thallium)

- electron beam computed tomography (EBCT)—to identify and measure calcium buildup in and around the coronary arteries indicative of coronary artery disease.

Analysis of blood sugar levels, a lipid profile to check cholesterol and triglyceride levels, and other tests also may be done to aide in the diagnosis of CAD.

5.6 TREATMENT

Treatments for CAD include lifestyle changes, medications, and special procedures to:

- relieve symptoms, if any,
- slow or stop, and possibly reverse, the atherosclerotic process by controlling or reducing modifiable risk factors
- lower the risk for blood clots forming which can cause a heart attack (myocardial infarction)

- dilate (widen) or bypass stenosed (narrowed) arteries
- reduce cardiac events such as arrhythmias, myocardial infarction, etc..

5.6.1 Lifestyle Changes

Lifestyle changes—everyone with CAD needs to make major lifestyle changes which include:
- adopting a more healthy lifestyle
- consuming a healthy diet to prevent or reduce high blood pressure and high blood cholesterol/triglycerides, and maintain a healthy weight
- stopping smoking/minimizing secondhand smoke
- using alcohol only in moderation or abstain entirely
- engaging in an appropriate daily physical activity/aerobic exercise
- achieving and maintaining normal weight
- reducing stress

For some individuals with CAD, these lifestyle changes may be the only treatment needed. For others more rigorous lifestyle changes may be needed.

5.6.2 Medical Treatment

Medications are needed in certain cases, in addition to making lifestyle changes. Some medications decrease the workload on the heart and relieve symptoms. Others decrease the chance of having a heart attack (myocardial infarction), or sudden death, and prevent or delay the need for a special procedure such as angioplasty or bypass surgery. Medications used to treat CAD may include:

- anticoagulants such as warfarin to "thin the blood" and prevent clots from forming in the arteries and blocking blood flow
- antiplatelet medications such as aspirin to prevent platelets from sticking/clumping together to form clots. Aspirin may be given to people who have had a heart attack, have angina, or who experience angina after angioplasty, to prevent recurrence
- ACE inhibitors such as enalapril to lower blood pressure, and reduce the strain on the heart and prevent a future heart attack
- beta blockers such as atenolol to slow heart rate and lower blood pressure in order to decrease the workload on the heart. Beta blockers are used to relieve angina and reduce the risk of a future heart attack
- calcium channel blockers to relax blood vessels and lower blood pressure and reduce the heart's workload, help keep coronary arteries open, and relieve and control angina
- nitroglycerin to prevent or relieve angina or chest discomfort
- nitrates (long acting) to open up the arteries to the heart, increase blood flow to the heart muscle and relieve chest pain/discomfort. Long acting nitrates can limit the occurrence of chest pain when used regularly over a long period.
- statins such as atorvastin to "normalize" cholesterol/triglycerides
- thrombolytics, such as activase to dissolve clots that can occur during heart attacks. Since around half the deaths occur in the first 1–2 hours, if a heart attack is suspected, one needs to get to a hospital as soon as possible in order to receive thrombolytic therapy, etc., if indicated.

Additional information on medical treatment is available at:

•   National Heart Lung Blood Institute
    How is a Heart Attack Treated
    http://www.nhlbi.nih.gov/dci/Diseases/HeartAttack/HeartAttack_
    treatments.html

5.6.3 Surgical Treatment

Under certain circumstances, special (invasive) procedures may be indicated, namely angioplasty and/or coronary artery bypass:

•   angioplasty to open blocked or stenosed (narrowed) coronary arteries to improve blood flow to the heart, relieve chest pain, and prevent a heart attack. Also, a stent may be placed in the affected artery to keep it open after the procedures.

•   coronary artery bypass surgery uses arteries or veins from other areas of the body to bypass an area(s) of a diseased/blocked coronary artery(s). This procedure improves blood flow to the affected heart muscle/tissue, relieves chest pain/discomfort, and may prevent a future heart attack.

Angioplasty or bypass surgery may be used to treat CAD when:

•   lifestyle changes and/or medications have not improved symptoms/ the disease process

•   symptoms/the disease process are worsening in spite of the "best" medical treatment feasible under the circumstances

Some individuals may need to have angioplasty or bypass surgery on an emergency basis during a heart attack to limit damage to the heart.

5.6.4 Cardiac Rehabilitation

Cardiac rehabilitation (rehab) may be prescribed by a doctor for angina, or after angioplasty, bypass surgery, or a heart attack. Together with medical and surgical treatment, cardiac rehab speeds recovery and development of a healthier lifestyle. Most people with CAD can benefit from rehab which often begins in the hospital after a heart attack, heart surgery or after heart treatment. Rehab usually continues on an outpatient basis after hospitalization for a specified period of time.

The cardiac rehab team may include:
- doctors (family doctor, heart specialist, surgeon)
- nurses
- exercise specialists
- physical therapists
- occupational therapists
- dieticians
- psychologists/behavior therapists

Rehab usually is composed of two parts:
- training to help one learn how to exercise properly and safely, strengthen muscles, and improve stamina. Exercise plans are based on individual ability, needs, and interests
- education, counseling, and training provide understanding regarding the heart condition and ways to reduce risk of future heart problems. The cardiac rehab team helps one learn how to cope with the stress of adjusting to a new lifestyle and how to deal with fears and expectations about the future.

Additional information on cardiac rehab programs is available at:

- American Heart Association
  Doctors Should Encourage Cardiac Rehab Programs
  http://www.americanheart.org/presenter.jhtml?identifier=302835

5.7 PREVENTION

Preventing CAD begins with knowing which risk factors are present and taking necessary action to modify them appropriately. The chances of developing CAD increases with the number of risk factors present and the action taken to modify them. By controlling your risk factors with lifestyle changes and medications, development of CAD may be prevented or at least slowed significantly reducing the risk of complications such as:

- myocardial ischemia and angina
- heart attack and permanent damage to the heart
- an arrhythmia (irregular heart beats) and consequences thereof
- heart failure
- sudden cardiac death

By staying as healthy as possible, risk for CAD and its complications can be lowered. Additional information is available at:

- National Heart Lung and Blood Institute
  What is Coronary Artery Disease
  http://www.nhlbi.nih.gov/health/dci/Diseases/Cad/CAD_WhatIs.html
  How Can I Prevent Coronary Artery Disease
  http://www.nhlbi.nih.gov/health/dci/Diseases/Cad/CAD_Prevention.html

CHAPTER 6

▼

PERIPHERAL ARTERY DISEASE

6.1 INTRODUCTION

Peripheral artery disease (PAD) occurs when diseased arteries in the legs become narrow (stenosed) or blocked (thrombosed) due to the buildup of fatty deposits/atherosclerosis.

PAD is reported to affect around 12 million persons in the United States. It affects over 4% of adults over age 40 and over 14 percent of adults 70 and older. African Americans are more than twice as likely to have PAD as Caucasians. It results in many thousands of leg amputations, many of which can be prevented with proper early recognition and treatment.

6.2 SYMPTOMS/SIGNS

The most common complaint of patients with PAD is intermittent claudication. This is a condition brought about by ischemia (lack of sufficient blood flow and oxygenation of tissues) of the leg muscles due to sclerosis and narrowing of the arteries of the legs characterized by intermittent attacks of cramping of calf muscles, lameness and pain on walking, chiefly affecting the calf muscles.

6.3 RISK FACTORS

Major risk factors for PAD are essentially the same as for atherosclerosis and include:

- other manifestations of atherosclerosis such as coronary artery disease
- diabetes mellitus
- hyperlipidemia
- hypertension
- sedentary lifestyle
- hyperhomocysteinemia

More than 95 percent of people with PAD have had one or more traditional major cardiovascular risk factors.

6.4 DIAGNOSIS

The earlier the diagnosis can be made and risk factors modified, the more likely prevention can be accomplished. Significant numbers of physicians routinely do not obtain a relevant history for PAD—and may overlook indications of the disease on physical examination or fail to promote preventive strategies.

Screening based on the ankle brachial index (ABI) using Doppler ultrasonagraphy, is a useful way to help diagnose patients with early PAD who may not have classic symptoms of claudication. Normally the ratio of blood pressure in the arms (brachial) versus the segments of the leg from the thigh to the ankle is around 1.0. In PAD the ratio becomes increasingly less than 1.0 in the affected leg. Segmental blood pressure measurements in the legs can reveal evidence for the existence of PAD.

Special attention to the pulses in the legs and feet, auscultation for leg arterial bruits, inspection of skin for postural color changes, and skin temperature may be almost as informative as an ABI evaluation. Together these evaluations and other procedures, when necessary, help to make the diagnosis.

6.5 MEDICAL TREATMENT

Medical treatment for prevention of PAD and complications thereof, revolves around modification of major risk factors and the use of diet, exercise and available medications. Patients with PAD should make every attempt to modify all existing risk factors regardless of the absence or severity of symptoms.

Smoking, a very important risk factor is correlated closely with developing PAD and intermittent claudication—more so than any other risk factor. Smoking cessation/avoiding secondhand smoke not only improves maximal treadmill walking distance, it also reduces the severity of the claudication. In addition, smoking cessation also appears to reduce the progression of PAD as shown by lower rates of claudication at rest, and amputation of the extremities, myocardial infarction, and death from other vascular causes.

Tight diabetic control may reduce the occurrence and progression of PAD, intermittent claudication, critical leg ischemia, limb infection, and amputation. Thus, glycemic (blood sugar) control in diabetics is considered central to PAD prevention and treatment.

Hypertension also is a major risk factor for PAD and its progression. Clinical studies support aggressive treatment of hypertension in patients with PAD. While the use of beta blocking drugs to control hypertension may decrease blood flow in the legs, such drugs are considered to be reasonably safe except in patients most severely affected with PAD.

Several large clinical trials have demonstrated the benefits of lipid lowering agents in patients with PAD, especially those with coexisting coronary or cerebral artery disease. Lipid lowering drugs have been shown to reduce PAD progression and the severity of claudication. Statin drugs and/or niacin are regarded as useful for this purpose.

A high serum homocysteine level also is reported to be an independent risk factor for PAD. Diets high in B vitamins and folate (as well as certain dietary supplements) lower elevated serum homocysteine levels effectively in most patients. However, it remains to be determined if doing so is beneficial for preventing/treating PAD.

A walking program is reported to be very helpful in treating PAD and relieving claudication.

Antiplatelet agents such as aspirin and clopidrogel, etc. have been found to be efficacious in improving claudication, walking distance, and stenosis of leg arteries in patients with PAD. Aspirin, in doses up to 325 mg/day generally is considered to be the antiplatelet drug of first choice. Aspirin alone given long term may beneficially modify the natural history and intermittent claudication symptoms.

6.6 SURGICAL TREATMENT

When leg arteries are blocked (stenosed) sufficiently, one may need surgical angioplasty to open them up. When this is done, a stent may be left in the affected artery to help keep it "open". Also, in certain cases, bypass surgery of the blocked/stenosed artery may be done. In more severe cases, when the affected limb cannot be "saved" and gangrene occurs, amputation may be required.

Additional information on PAD is available at:
- American Academy of Family Physicians
  Peripheral Artery Disease and Claudication
  http://www.familydoctor.org/008.xml?xml
  Management of Peripheral Arterial Disease
  http://www.aafp.org/afp/20040201/525.html
- American Heart Association
  What is Peripheral Vascular Disease
  http://www.americanheart.org/presenter.jhtml?identifier=4692
- Johns Hopkins Bloomberg School of Public Health
  High Burden of Peripheral Artery Disease
  http://www.jhsph.edu/PublicHealthNews/articles/Selvin_PAD.html

CHAPTER 7

▼

HYPERTENSION

7.1 INTRODUCTION

Hypertension (high blood pressure) constitutes one of the most important public health problems in the developed countries of the world including the United States. It is very common in occurrence, usually asymptomatic in its early stages, and easily detectable and treatable. Untreated, hypertension often leads to other CVD and lethal complications.

Around 40–50 million Americans are estimated to have hypertension and another 40 million or so, prehypertension. Only about 50 percent of those with hypertension currently are being treated and around 50 percent of these are regarded as having inadequately controlled hypertension. Reasons given for this rather poor record to date include such things as:

- many patients are largely asymptomatic and do not see the need for therapy and become non-compliant with the doctor's treatment program

- mechanism(s) underlying the high blood pressure in any given case is not fully understood and appropriate drug therapy/treatment is not administered
- lifelong treatment is usually required and individuals "cannot see the light at the end of the tunnel" and give up and drop out of treatment
- therapy causes side effects which cause the patient to stop taking pre-scribed medication/treatment

Although our understanding of the pathophysiology of hypertension has increased significantly, in 90 to 95 percent of cases, the cause(s) (and thus potentially the best means of prevention or treatment) is still largely unknown.

7.2 CLASSIFICATION

There are five generally recognized categories of classification of blood pressure. These are:

- Normal   <120 systolic/<80 diastolic
- Prehypertension   120–139 systolic/80–89 diastolic
- Stage 1 hypertension   140–159 systolic/90–99 diastolic
- Stage 2 hypertension   >160 systolic/>100 diastolic
- Isolated systolic hypertension*   >140 systolic/<90 diastolic

* occurs mostly in individuals over 55 years of age

While the above classification is generally considered to be useful for prognosis and treatment, it should be noted that risk of complications from hypertension increases in a continuous graded manner for increases in both systolic and diastolic pressures.

7.3. Risk Factors

Individuals at risk for developing hypertension include those having:

- African or Native American ancestry
- excessive alcohol intake
- a stressful lifestyle
- a family history of hypertension
- insufficient potassium intake and/or excess sodium intake in the diet
- low dietary consumption of fruits and vegetables
- overweight/obesity
- prehypertension (high "normal" blood pressure)
- sedentary life style
- a smoking habit

7.4 Diagnosis

Hypertension is diagnosed with a cuff sphygmomanometer. Blood pressure needs to be checked at regular intervals starting early in life in order to diagnose high blood pressure in its early stages to more easily prevent complication/serious outcomes. Most doctors diagnose high blood pressure on the basis of readings taken on more than one, and usually several occasions. A consistent reading of 140/90 or higher is generally considered to be high blood pressure. Consistent readings of 120–139 systolic/80–89 diastolic generally are regarded as prehypertension, a risk factor for subsequent development of hypertension.

Some individuals have high blood pressure readings only when visiting a doctor's office. This condition is regarded as being due largely to emotional stress and is called "white coat hypertension". If a doctor suspects that this may be the case, it may be necessary to monitor blood pressure at home with the patient wearing a device called an ambulatory blood pressure monitor for 24 hours which takes blood pressure readings every 30 minutes or so. When blood pressure is found to be elevated only in the doctor's office and not at home the diagnosis of white-coat hypertension may be made and handled accordingly.

While various patient populations all tend to show a progressive rise in blood pressure with age, proportions with abnormal elevations vary considerably from population to population. Women tend to have slightly lower blood pressure than men in the third and fourth decade and slightly higher blood pressure thereafter.

7.5 PATHOPHYSIOLOGY

Although our understanding of the pathophysiology of hypertension has increased dramatically over past decades, in essential hypertension, which represents over 90 percent of all cases of high blood pressure, tends to cluster in families but the cause remains largely unknown. Multiple genes likely are involved in the pathogenesis and give rise to a number of inherited biochemical abnormalities leading to essential hypertension.

Secondary hypertension (high blood pressure in which a correctable cause can be found) represents less than 10 percent of all cases of hypertension. Correctable causes may include such things as:

- renal artery stenosis from atherosclerosis, etc.
- coarctation of the aorta
- thyroid disease producing excess thyroid hormones(s)
- Cushing's disease of the adrenals

- pheochromocytoma
- drugs (such as alcohol, oral contraceptives, steroids, amphetamines, cocaine, and non steroidal anti-inflammatory agents, etc.)

Most patients with hypertension are asymptomatic, especially in the early stages of the disease. In cases of accelerated essential hypertension or secondary hypertension, symptoms generally are related to target organs involved, namely brain, eyes, kidneys, heart and peripheral arteries.

Further discussion of secondary hypertension lies outside the scope of this book. For further information, the reader may consult various Web resources and corresponding websites found in the Author's List, Chapter 10.

7.6 HYPERTENSION AND CVD

High blood pressure represents only one of several proven major modifiable risk factors for CVD. Together, these risk factors provide a strong basis for predicting overall CVD risk and complications. Elevated blood pressure increases morbidity and mortality from atherosclerosis, carotid artery disease, cerebral artery disease/stroke, coronary artery disease, myocardial infarction, peripheral artery disease, congestive heart failure, and end stage renal disease.

Individuals with a low CVD risk profile (serum cholesterol level <200 mg/dl, blood pressure <120/80 mmHg and no current smoking) are reported to have a 72–85 percent lower mortality from CVD and a 40–58 percent lower mortality from all causes compared with those who have one or more of these three modifiable risk factors. The greater life expectancy for low risk individuals ranges from 5.8 to 9.5 years. Computer programs and risk calculating charts are available to assist in determining risk.

7.7 Prevention/Treatment

Essential hypertension can be prevented. If it occurs, it can be treated successfully in most cases. The ultimate goal of treatment is to normalize blood pressure.

Lifestyle interventions are the cornerstone of both prevention and treatment, and are more likely to be successful, and the absolute reduction in the risk for hypertension to be greater, when targeted individuals are older or have a higher risk of developing hypertension. Also, prevention strategies applied early in life provide the greatest long term potential for controlling modifiable risk factors that lead to hypertension and its complications.

Lowering sodium content and calories from food, weight control, exercise, abstinence or moderation in alcohol intake, increased potassium intake in the diet, smoking cessation, and eating a diet rich in fruits and vegetables can prevent hypertension and even result in a significant improvement in high blood pressure, once hypertension has occurred.

Lifestyle modifications considered most effective in the primary prevention and/or treatment of hypertension include:
- adopting a healthy lifestyle
- mediating, engaging in mindfulness
- engaging in a regular aerobic level of physical activity 30–60 minutes (preferably 60) per day, 5–7 (preferably 7) days per week, such as a brisk 3 mile walk daily

- achieving/maintaining normal body weight (body mass index less than 25)
- limiting alcohol consumption to no more than 1–2 alcoholic drinks per day in men and 1 in women
- reducing dietary sodium intake to no more than 2400 mg per day (6 grams of sodium chloride)
- consuming a diet rich in fruits and vegetables, 5 to 9 (preferably 9) servings per day, low fat dairy products, and having a reduced content of saturated and total fat
- using a DASH (dietary approaches to stop hypertension) type eating plan
- reducing stress/increasing coping
- smoking cessation/avoiding secondhand smoke

Lifestyle interventions considered to be uncertain or of less proven efficacy for primary prevention and/or treatment of hypertension include:
- calcium supplementation—this appears to result in only a small reduction in blood pressure. However, adequate calcium intake of 1,000 to 1,200 mg per day remains prudent for good health in general
- fish oil supplementation—in high doses, fish oil lowers blood pressure only slightly in hypertensive patients
- herbal or botanical supplements—there are no well controlled clinical studies supporting the efficacy of such products in the prevention and/or treatment of hypertension

Smoking injures blood vessel walls and speeds up the process of hardening of the arteries. This applies even to filtered cigarettes. Even though smoking does not cause high blood pressure directly, it is bad for anyone, especially those with high blood pressure. If you don't smoke, don't start. If you smoke, quit. Once you quit, your risk of having a heart or stroke is reduced markedly.

Smoking by women in the United States causes almost as many deaths from heart disease as from lung cancer. If a woman smokes, she is 2 to 6 times more likely to suffer a heart attack, and the risk increases with the number of cigarettes smoked each day. Smoking also boosts the risk of stroke. Quitting smoking cuts the risk of a heart attack dramatically by more than 50 percent and also reduces the risk of a second heart attack in someone who has had one.

The demonstrated reductions in blood pressure using appropriate lifestyle interventions can be as large as those seen with antihypertensive medications and can be sustained long term.

A wide variety of FDA approved, effective antihypertensive drugs are now available. For additional information, see the Food and Drug Administration reference/website at the end of this section.

Guidelines for consideration in the treatment of high blood pressure recently issued by the National Heart Lung Blood Institute include the following:

- in those older than age 50, systolic blood pressure (BP) of greater than 140 mmHg is a more important CVD risk factor than diastolic BP
- beginning at 115/75 mmHg, CVD risk doubles for each increment of 20/10 mmHg

- those who are normotensive at 55 years of age will have a 90 percent lifetime risk of developing hypertension
- prehypertensive individuals (systolic 120–39 mmHg or diasystolic BP of 80–89 mmHg) require health-promoting lifestyle modifications to prevent the progressive rise in BP and CVD
- for uncomplicated hypertension, a thiazide diuretic should be used in drug treatment for most people, either alone or combined with drugs from other classes
- specific high-risk conditions are compelling indications for the use of other antihypertensive drug classes (angiotension converting enzyme inhibitors, angiotenson-receptor blockers, beta blockers, calcium channel blockers)
- two or more antihypertensive medications will be required to achieve goal BP (<149/90 mmHg or 130/80 mmHg) for patients with diabetes and chronic kidney disease
- for patients whose BP is more than 20 mmHg above the systolic goal or more than 10 mmHg above the diasystolic BP goal, initiation of therapy using two agents, one of which is usually a thiazide diuretic, should be considered
- regardless of therapy or care, hypertension will be controlled only if patients are motivated to stay on their treatment plan

Additional information on hypertension is available at:
- American Heart Association
  High Blood Pressure
  http://www.americanheart.org/presenter.jhml?identifier=2114

- Food and Drug Administration
  Lessening the Pressure; Array of Drugs Tames Hypertension
  http://www.fda.gov/fdac/features/1999/499_hbp.html
- National Heart Lung and Blood Institute
  DASH Eating Plan
  http://www.nhlbi.nih.gov/health/public/heart/hbp/dash
  Primary Prevention of Hypertension
  http://www.nhlbi.nih.gov/health/prof/heart/hbp/pphbp.htm
  Prevention, Detection, Evaluation and Treatment of High Blood Pressure
  http://www.nhlbi.nih.gov/guidelines/hypertension/jnc7full.pdf
  Risk Assessment Tool for Estimating Your 10-Year Risk of Having a Heart Attack
  http://hin.nhlbi.gov/atpiii/calculator.asp?usetype=pub
  Quit Smoking
  http://www.nhlbi.nih.gov/hbp/prevent/q_smoking/q_smoke.htm

CHAPTER 8

▼

MODIFIABLE CVD RISK FACTORS

8.1 INTRODUCTION

The risk of CVD rises as people age, and men tend to develop CVD much earlier in life than women. More specifically, men age 45 and older are considered to be at increased risk for CVD, while women 55–65 and older share a similar increased risk due to age. A woman's female hormones are regarded as giving a level of protection from CVD before menopause.

Thus, CVD presents in women an average of 10 years or later in life than men. However, after menopause, woman develop CVD as often as men, and women who do so, don't fare as well as men. In fact, women are more likely to die from CVD then men. Although CVD is the leading cause of death for both adult men and women, many do not realize that this is the case, or that CVD is preventable.

In general, most experts believe that the best way to prevent or combat CVD is to know one's risk factors, "own" them, and fully address and treat those that are modifiable for the better—and profit accordingly.

Unfortunately, while many individuals may be able to rattle off one or more of the CVD risk factors, they frequently fail to "internalize" them as such and be able to say—that's a significant risk factor(s) for me—therefore I am at risk for CVD and I am going to do something constructive about it now!

Rather, Americans have become complacent about CVD and overestimate the status of their cardiovascular health. For example, around 75 percent or so say they try to maintain a healthy weight but only around one third do so. In addition, around two thirds say they try to exercise regularly but only around 20 percent do so. And around 60 percent say they try to avoid high fat, high cholesterol foods whereas only around 10 percent follow dietary guidelines established by the American Heart Association or Dietary Guidelines for Americans. In addition, some 60 percent or so of individuals queried do not believe they are at much risk for CVD, and a similar percentage of people just do not believe CVD is the "killer disease" that it is reported to be.

In spite of the aforementioned public opinions, it is important to recognize that there are a number of significant established risk factors for CVD. They are typically labeled modifiable (controllable) and unmodifiable (uncontrollable). And, prevention of CVD is accomplished by controlling/treating modifiable risk factors for the better.

Because of advances in medicine, individuals with CVD are living longer and more productive lives than ever before. Dramatic reductions in CVD have occurred over the past few decades, and prevention measures are still the best weapon in the fight against CVD in order to bring about further reductions.

However, as with anything in life, there are no guarantees. Whether one is healthy now, or at moderate to high risk for CVD, or has "survived" a form of CVD, the best approach is still essentially the same—protect yourself by acknowledging, correcting and minimizing all modifiable CVD risk factors you may have or develop over time.

Therefore, controlling modifiable risk factors is regarded as the most effective way of decreasing CVD. Modifiable risk factors include:

- air pollution
- alcohol intake
- C-reactive protein
- cholesterols/triglycerides
  - high total cholesterol
  - low HDL
  - high LDL
  - high triglycerides
- diabetes mellitus
- hyperhomocysteinemia
- hypertension
- kidney disease
- metabolic syndrome x
- oral contraceptives
- overweight/obesity
- oxidative stress
- periodontal disease

- psychological stress
- sedentary lifestyle
- smoking/secondhand smoke

Each of the above modifiable risk factors has its own importance for CVD and will be discussed individually in order to provide a better understanding and basis for remedial action for consideration.

8.2 AIR POLLUTION

Air pollution is regarded as a modifiable risk factor for the development of CVD. The Environmental Protection Agency (EPA) has indicated that "tens of thousands of people die each year from breathing tiny particles in the environment (polluted air)". Death rates in the 90 largest US cities rise by 0.5 percent with only a very small increase—10 micrograms per cubic meter—in particles less than 10 micrometers in diameter. And, the combined long-term effect of such air pollution has been estimated to reach as much as 60,000 deaths each year, many from CVD, due to such particulate matter.

Air pollution is composed of a number of environmental factors such as carbon monoxide, nitrates, sulfur dioxide, ozone, lead, secondhand tobacco smoke, and particulate matter. Vehicle emissions, tire fragmentation, road dust, power generation and industrial combustion, smelting/metal processing, construction, demolition activities, residential wood burning, windblown soil, pollens, molds, forest fires, volcanic emissions, and sea spray also all produce particulate matter air pollution.

Risk Factors for CVD

While it long has been known that people in more air polluted areas die earlier from CVD, the increase in relative risk for cardiovascular disease due to air pollution for any given individual is regarded as not as large as the impact of major risk factors such as high blood pressure or elevated blood cholesterol levels. However, air pollution remains a serious public health problem due to the enormous number of people affected and because exposure to air pollution occurs over an entire lifetime, especially in the cities. In addition, higher concentrations of air particle pollution in cities continues to result in increased hospital admissions for CVD.

Air pollution also is now known to produce chronic oxidative (metabolic) stress in the body and accelerate the atherosclerotic process basis for CVD.

Secondhand smoke

Secondhand smoke is regarded as the single largest contributor to indoor air pollution when a smoker is present. Studies indicate that secondhand smoke significantly adversely affects the heart and circulatory system leading to CVD. Exposure to the secondhand smoke of just one cigarette per day is reported to accelerate the atherosclerotic process. Thus, protecting oneself from secondhand smoke is critical in avoiding CVD.

Traffic Exhaust

Exposure to traffic-related air pollutants has been found to be more highly related to mortality from CVD than city-wide background levels. And, individuals who live near a major roadway are more likely to die of a cardiovascular event such as a heart attack.

Carbon Monoxide

Carbon monoxide (CO) is a colorless, odorless and highly poisonous gas and common pollutant associated with combustion reactions, and especially found in exhaust from cars, trucks, and other vehicles, as well as in cigarette smoke. With increasing CO blood levels, the level of oxygen that blood can carry is decreased due to the formation of carboxyhemoglobin. At any significant level, CO is harmful to the body and even deadly at high levels. Thus, smoking tobacco and breathing secondhand environmental smoke raises CO levels in blood leading to CVD. At 20 ppm of CO in blood there is a very significant loss of oxygen carried by blood to vital organs such as the heart and brain. An average person who smokes one pack a day of cigarettes can have a blood CO level up to 20 ppm and more, and someone who smokes two packs per day may have a blood CO level of up to 40 PPM and higher. When smoking stops, blood CO levels usually return to normal in a few days.

Treatment goals

Individuals should avoid as many different kinds, and as much of, air pollution as possible in order to minimize the risk of CVD.

Additional information on air pollution and CVD is available at:
*   American Heart Association
    Air Pollution, Heart Disease and Stroke
    http://www.americanheart.org/presenter.jhtml?identifier=4419

Air Pollution, Even at "Safe" Levels, is Bad for the Heart
http://www.americanheart.org/presenter.jhtml?identifier=3016889

Information on EPA (Environmental Protection Agency) Air Quality Index and CVD is available at: http://www.epa.gov/airnow/aqibroch.aqi. html

8.3 ALCOHOL

For many centuries, individuals have consumed fermented beverages and have been discussing whether drinking alcohol is "good" or "bad". And, it has been discovered that the difference is largely in the amount consumed—in moderate amounts, it may be beneficial to health whereas heavy drinking is a major cause of preventable CVD disease, disability, and death. In the United States, heavy drinking may be involved in around 50 percent of fatal traffic accidents and can cause CVD disease as well as cancer and other serious health problems.

The upper boundary of moderate drinking is regarded as the point at which the health benefits of alcohol clearly outweigh the risks. The latest consensus of opinion defines this point at up to one to two drinks per day for men and no more than one drink per day for women. One drink may be defined as 12 ounces of beer, 5 ounces of wine, or 1.5 ounces of hard liquor such as scotch, gin or whisky. Each of these servings has around 12 to 14 grams of alcohol. These parameters are the ones used by the Dietary Guidelines for Americans and are widely used in the United States.

CVD Health Benefits of Alcohol

Many clinical studies have demonstrated the health benefits from moderate consumption of alcohol in terms of reduction in risk for carotid artery disease, cerebral artery disease, coronary artery disease, myocardial infarction, ischemic stroke, peripheral artery disease, sudden cardiac death, and death from all CVD causes. This reduction in risk for CVD has been observed in both men and women, and applies not only to those with no apparent, as well as those with, CVD.

The benefits of moderate alcohol consumption are found to be reasonably consistent from study to study, and range from a 25 to 40 percent reduction in CVD risk. Moderate drinking may not only help prevent CVD but also protect against type 2 diabetes mellitus. Alcohol (ethanol) is reported to affect levels of lipids (cholesterol and triglycerides) and insulin in the blood as well as inflammation in the body and coagulation of blood (clotting).

Moderate alcohol consumption is believed to protect against CVD in a number of ways, namely:

- raising HDL or "good" cholesterol which in turn is regarded as associated with greater protection against CVD
- favorably influencing blood clotting factors, such as tissue type plasminogen activator, fibrinogen, clotting factor VII, and Willebrand factor. These beneficial effects of alcohol tend to prevent the formation of blood clots that can block arteries in the heart, neck and brain, the cause of many heart attacks and strokes.

The benefits and risks of moderate drinking change over a lifetime. Generally, risks exceed benefits until middle age, when CVD begins to account for an increasingly large share of the burden of disease and death.

Whether or not to drink or continue drinking alcohol, especially for health purposes can only be answered by a physician/healthcare provider for each individual case. However, if one doesn't drink there is no need to start since similar CVD benefits can be obtained with diet, exercise and other measures.

Additional information on alcohol is available at:
• Harvard School of Public Health
   Alcohol
   http://www.hsph.harvard.edu/nutritionsource/alcohol.html

Adverse CVD Effects of Alcohol

While moderate alcohol consumption may be regarded as having certain CVD health benefits, excessive consumption of alcohol is associated with at least 4 types of CVDs, namely:
• alcoholic cardiomyopathy
• alcoholic hemorrhagic stroke
• atherosclerotic CVD
• secondary hypertension

Both atherosclerotic CVD and secondary hypertension have been discussed previously. Therefore, discussion in this section will be limited to alcoholic cardiomyopathy and hemorrhagic stroke.

Alcoholic cardiomyopathy

Around one third of chronic alcoholic men and women have been found to suffer from alcoholic cardiomyopathy. In this condition the heart is in failure, is dilated and the ejection fraction (measure of the heart's ability to pump sufficient blood with each beat) is depressed. These adverse effects on the heart are correlated with total lifetime intake of alcohol. The threshold dose for development of cardiomyopathy is considerably less in women (only 60 percent) than in men. This indicates that women are more sensitive than men for the development of alcoholic cardiomyopathy.

Treatment of alcoholic cardiomyopathy consists of a program fostering abstinence from alcohol along with a healthy lifestyle.

Additional information is available at:
- Texas Heart Institute
  Cardiomyopathy
  http://www.texasinstitute.org/dilated.html

Alcoholic Hemorrhagic Stroke

Excessive alcohol consumption is associated with hemorrhagic stroke. Heavy consumption of alcohol leads to an elevation of blood pressure which is associated with hemorrhagic stroke. However, clinical studies have shown a significant influence of excessive alcohol intake even after adjustment for blood pressure effects—especially for strokes due to intracerebral hemorrhage and subarachnoid hemorrhage. Alcohol intoxication preceding a subarachnoid hemorrhage is reported to be two to four times as common in males and three to five times as common in females.

The risk of a hemorrhagic stroke is reported to increase linearly with an increase of blood gamma glutamyltransferase (gamma GT), a blood enzyme indicator of excessive alcohol consumption.

CVD and stroke due to excessive alcohol intake (alcoholism) remains preventable through abstention and/or moderation in alcohol consumption and the adoption of a more healthy lifestyle.

Additional information on alcoholic hemorrhagic stroke is available at:
* National Institute of Neurological Disorders and Stroke
  What You Need to Know About Stroke
  http://www.ninds.nih.gov/disorders/stroke/stroke_needtoknow.htm

8.4 C-Reactive Protein (CRP)

Inflammation, a process whereby the body responds to injury, releasing a number of chemical agents into the circulation, is an important factor in the development of atherosclerosis/cardiovascular diseases (CVDs).

C-Reactive Protein (CRP) is one of the proteins released into the circulation that is increased during inflammation in the body. Thus, measuring blood levels of CRP has recently become accepted as a new and important way to assess CVD risk. And, more recently, a high sensitivity (hs) assay for CRP (known as hs-CRP) has now become widely available for determining CVD risk.

AHA/CDC CRP Risk Categories

The AHA (American Heart Association) and CDC (Centers for Disease Control and Prevention) defines CVD risk groups using the hs-CRP blood test levels as follows:

- low risk—less than 1.0 mg (milligram)/L (liter)
- average risk—1.0 to 3.0 mg/L
- high risk—above 3.0 mg/L

Results generally are interpreted on such a relative scale where people with the highest values have the highest risk of CVD and those with the lowest values have the lowest risk.

CRP Interpretation

High levels of hs-CRP are reported to predict:

- new coronary events in patients with unstable angina and acute myocardial infarction (heart attack)
- lower survival rate from CVD events
- that a coronary artery will reclose after it has been opened by balloon angioplasty
- prognosis and recurrent events in patients with stroke and peripheral arterial disease
- overall CVD risk and progression in general.

Elderly men and women who have an elevated blood hs-CRP level are reported to have up to a 45 percent increase in their risk for CVD. Men predicted to have a 10 to 20 percent chance (intermediate risk) of having a coronary event over the next 10 years based on traditional risk factor assessment, were found to have an actual observed rate of 32 percent when they had elevated, high hs-CRP levels.

Women, on the other hand, who had a predicted CVD rate greater than 20 percent in 10 years, actually had about a 31 percent chance of having a heart attack or dying of heart disease when they had a hs-CRP level in the high risk category. And, when their CRP indicates low CVD risk, coronary events actually occur in the 16 percent range.

In the Women's Health Study, CRP levels even proved to be a better predictor of future CVD events than elevated LDL cholesterol levels. Based on the results of this study, it has been proposed that a combined evaluation of CRP and LDL may prove superior in predicting CVD risk because these two tests appear to complement each other. In addition, it should be remembered that many individuals who have a CVD event such as a heart attack, have LDL cholesterol levels below 130 milligrams per deciliter (mg/dl).

It may not be discernable in any given case what may be causing low-grade chronic inflammation that appears to put otherwise "healthy" people at risk for CVD. Possible subclinical infections such as periodontitis, chlamydia (sexually transmitted bacteria) helicobacter pylori (cause of ulcers), herpes simplex, or cytomegalovirus may be involved. In addition, cancer, autoimmune disease, and arthritis also may be involved in the atherosclerotic inflammatory process and elevation of CRP.

In general, if a person's global CVD assessment is low (in other words, the possibility of developing CVD is less than 10 percent in 10 years) no CRP test is immediately warranted.

When a person's global risk score is in the intermediate range (10 to 20 percent), a hs-CRP test may help predict a cardiovascular or stroke event, and help direct further evaluation and therapy.

However, when a person has a global high risk score (greater than 20 percent in 10 years), or has established heart disease or stroke, intensive treatment regardless of hs-CRP levels may be considered to be in order.

Treatment Goal

Every effort should be made to determine what may be causing the low grade inflammatory response that may lead to elevated CRP levels and CVD in order that such may be treated appropriately, and hs-CRP reduced to low risk levels. However, it is not known if this will actually reduce CVD risk.

Additional information on CRP is available at:
- American Heart Association
  Inflammation, Heart Disease and Stroke: The Role of C-Reactive Protein
  http://www.americanheart.org/present.jhtml?identifier=4648
  AHA/CDC Panel Issues Recommendations on CRP Testing
  http://www.americanheart.org/present.jhtml?identifier=3007984
  CRP Improves CVD Risk Prediction in Metabolic Syndrome x
  http://www.americanheart.org/present.jhtml?identifier=3007985

- Lab Tests Online

  C-Reactive Protein (hs-CRP)

  http://www.labtestonlne.org/understanding/analytes/hscrp/test.html

8.5 CHOLESTEROL/TRIGLYCERIDES

The National Heart, Lung, and Blood Institute (NHBLI), American College of Cardiology (ACC) and the American Heart Association (AHA) update to the National Cholesterol Education Program (NCEP) clinical practice guidelines on cholesterol management advises physicians to consider new, more intensive treatment options for people at high and moderately high risk for CVD, a heart attack or stroke, etc. The document is based on a review of 5 major clinical trials of statin therapy conducted since the previous NCEP cholesterol guidelines known as the Adult Treatment Panel (ATP) III Report. NHLBI, a component of the National Institutes of Health, coordinates the NCEP.

The recent clinical trials add to the evidence that when one considers LDL ("bad") cholesterol, lower is better for persons with high risk for a heart attack or stroke. These trials show a direct relationship between lower LDL cholesterol levels and reduced risk of CVD.

NCEP Recommendations

NCEP recommends that the following blood cholesterol levels be achieved:

- high and very high risk
  - high risk: LDL <100 mg/dl
  - very high risk: LDL <70 mg/dl

For very high risk patients whose LDL levels are already below 100 mg/dl, there is the option to use drug therapy to reach the goal of <70 mg/dl.

For the overall category of high risk patients, the update lowers the threshold for drug therapy to an LDL of 100 mg/dl or less, and recommends drug therapy for those high risk patients whose LDL is 100 to 129 mg/l.

The NCEP defines high-risk patients as those who have coronary artery disease or disease of the blood vessels to the brain or extremities, diabetes, or multiple (2 or more) risk factors (e.g., smoking, hypertension) that give them a greater than 20 percent chance of having a heart attack within 10 years. Very high-risk patients are regarded as those who have CVD together with either multiple risk factors (especially diabetes), or severe and poorly controlled risk factors (e.g., continued smoking, or metabolic syndrome x (a constellation of risk factors associated with overweight/obesity including elevated triglycerides and blood pressure and low HDL). Patients hospitalized for acute coronary syndrome such as a heart attack also are at very high risk.

Moderately high risk patients are considered to be those who have multiple (2 or more) risk factors for coronary artery disease together with a 10 to 20 percent risk of a heart attack within 10 years. For moderately high risk patients, the goal remains an LDL under 130 mg/dl, however, the update provides a therapeutic option to set a lower LDL goal of under 100 mg/dl and to use drug therapy at LDL levels of 100–129 mg/dl to reach this lower goal.

For high risk or moderately high risk patients, the update advises that the intensity of LDL lowering drug therapy be sufficient to achieve at least a 30 percent reduction in LDL levels. This can be accomplished by taking a statin medication with other drugs (e.g., bile acid resins, nicotinic acid, etc.) or with food products containing plant stanol/sterols.

For moderate risk, recommendations were not revised in the update. This includes those with moderate risk (2 or more risk factors plus an under 10 percent risk of a heart attack in 10 years) or those with 0 to 1 risk factor. According to the update, the absolute benefits for people at the lower levels of risk are less clear cut and recent clinical trials do not suggest a modification of treatment goals and objectives.

Like the previous recommendation, the update addresses and emphasizes cholesterol lowering in older persons (age 65 or above). High risk older persons with established cardiovascular disease are included in the recommendations for intensive LDL-lowering therapy. Although the update suggests that physicians use their clinical judgment to determine whether intensive LDL lowering therapy is warranted in older persons, these people should not be excluded from the potential benefits of LDL lowering treatment just because of age.

An acceptable "normal" blood lipid profile for individuals with little or no risk for cardiovascular disease is reported to be as follows:
- total cholesterol (TC) < 200 mg/dl
- HDL cholesterol > 40 mg/dl
- LDL cholesterol < 130 mg/dl
- triglycerides <150 mg/dl

- TC/HDL ratio < 4

Therapeutic Lifestyle Goals

The published report emphasizes the importance of therapeutic lifestyle changes (TLC)—intensive use of nutrition, diet, physical activity, and weight control for optimal blood lipid management. As such, lifestyle changes continue to be an essential part of controlling blood lipid levels.

TLC is regarded as having the potential to reduce CVD risk through mechanisms beyond LDL lowering.

Additional information on cholesterol guidelines is available at:
- National Heart Lung Blood Institute
  Detection, Evaluation, and Treatment of High Blood Cholesterol in Adults (Adult Treatment Panel III)
  http://www.nhlbi.nih.gov/guidelines/cholesterol/index.htm

A 10 year heart attack risk calculator can be found at the website above.

8.6 DIABETES MELLITUS

Diabetes mellitus is a major risk factor for CVD. Uncontrolled blood sugar and lipid levels lead to diffuse endothelial disease and atherosclerotic damage to the arterial blood vessels throughout the body.

Risk for CVD

Diabetics are 2 to 4 times more likely than others to have a heart attack or a stroke. And, diabetics usually have a family member who has had diabetes and CVD as well, placing them in a known higher risk group for CVD.

Instead of having one or two CVD risk factors, diabetics usually have a collection, making them more prone to developing CVD. When certain risk factors occur together in one person, they may form a powerful health threat known as the metabolic syndrome x.

Metabolic syndrome x is very common among diabetics. Individuals with this disorder show high levels of a chemical in blood called plasminogen activator inhibitor-1 which is known to promote blood-clot formation. And a blood clot may trigger heart attack or stroke, and this may account for at least one of the reasons why diabetes is an important risk factor for CVD.

One of the greatest threats faced by people with diabetes is peripheral artery disease which increases the risk for amputation of a limb(s) due to inadequate circulation in the legs.

In addition, while smoking is not more common among diabetics, it is reported to be more dangerous in this group than in any other. If one has the metabolic syndrome x, smoking is reported to further increase the risk of CVD and death by about 40 percent.

Treatment goal

Life style changes usually are necessary to bring about satisfactory control in diabetes including diet, exercise, weight control, and medications when necessary in order to reduce risk for CVD.

Additional information is available at:
- National Institute of Diabetes and Digestive and Kidney Diseases
  The Link between Diabetes and Cardiovascular Disease
  http://www.niddk.nih.gov/diabetes/pubs/CVD_factsheet.pdf
  Be Smart About Your Heart: Control ABCs of Diabetes
  http://www.ndep.nih.gov/campagins/BeSmart/BeSmart_overview.htm

8.7 HOMOCYSTEINE

Homocysteine is a chemical found in blood that is produced when an amino acid, methionine, is metabolized (broken down) in the body. While we all have some homocysteine in our blood, elevated levels (also called hyperhomocysteinemia) may produce irritation of the endothelium of arteries increasing the risk for:
- atherosclerosis, carotid artery disease, coronary artery disease, peripheral artery disease, cerebral artery disease, myocardial infarction and stroke
- blood clots in the leg veins
- pulmonary embolism, a complication of deep venous thrombosis of the legs

Total plasma homocysteine increases with age, is higher in men than in women, and increases markedly with the number of cigarettes smoked daily in all age groups, particularly in women. Furthermore, total plasma homocysteine correlates directly with total cholesterol, blood pressure, and heart rate, and is inversely related to physical activity—sedentary individuals have higher blood homocysteine levels.

Elevated Homocysteine levels

Some people have elevated homocysteine levels caused by a deficiency of B vitamins and folate in their diet. And certain diseases such as kidney, thyroid, and psoriasis as well as medications such as antiepileptic drugs and methotrexate also may cause high blood homocysteine levels. Homocysteine blood levels also increase in women after the menopause. Some individuals may have a genetic mutation which may lead to elevated blood homocysteine levels.

Homocysteine is measured through a routine blood test. Occasionally, a methionine loading test is done in which homocysteine blood levels are measured before and after the intake of 100 mg/kg of methionine dissolved in orange juice. Individuals having a high risk of cardiovascular disease but normal baseline homocysteine blood levels may benefit most from this test. Those with an abnormal test result may respond better to vitamin B6 supplements compared with folic acid treatment. Generally speaking, a fasting blood homocysteine level less than 13 micromolar per liter (13 µmol/l) is considered normal, and over 13 µmol/l as elevated.

While an elevated blood homocysteine level is associated with an increased risk of developing CVD, the magnitude of the risk is not well defined.

However, individuals with an elevated blood homocysteine level appear to have about twice the risk of CVD events compared with those with a normal blood homocysteine level. And increasing levels of blood homocysteine appear to signify an additional rise in the risk. The length of time an individual has had elevated blood homocysteine levels also may increase risk accordingly.

Individuals with a genetic homocysteine disorder are prone to develop severe CVD in their teens and 20s. In these individuals, a defective enzyme causes accumulation of homocysteine in blood, putting them at risk for developing atherosclerosis and blood clots in the arteries and veins. While genetic hyperhomocysteinemia affects about 1 in 200,000, many more individuals appear to have milder or moderately elevated blood homocysteine levels.

Treatment

Elevated blood homocysteine levels can be lowered in most patients by increasing the dietary intake of folic acid and B vitamins or by consuming 5 to 9 servings of fruits and vegetables (especially green leafy vegetables). Good sources of folate include fortified breads, cereals, lentils, chickpeas, asparagus, spinach and most beans. If adjusting dietary intake does not lower blood homocysteine levels to normal, over the counter multivitamins or B complex vitamins may prove to be effective. If necessary, a doctor can prescribe appropriate medications that contain the necessary levels of folic acid/B vitamins to produce the desired result.

Considerable evidence now exists that hyperhomocysteinemia is strongly and independently related to atherosclerosis, carotid artery disease, cerebral artery disease/stroke, coronary artery disease, myocardial infarction, peripheral artery disease and venous thrombosis. On the basis of retrospective and prospective studies, it is now widely accepted that increased total blood plasma homocysteine is a risk factor for CVD and should be considered for treatment. However, further well controlled clinical trials are needed to determine whether lowering elevated blood plasma homocysteine levels actually decreases the risk for CVD and complications thereof.

Additional information on homocysteine and CVD is available at:

*   American Heart Association
    Homocysteine, Folic Acid and Cardiovascular Disease
    http://www.americanheart.org/presenter.jhtml?identifier=4677
    What is Homocysteine?
    http://www.americanheart.org/presenter.jhtml?identifier=535
    Elevated Homocysteine in Heart Patients Linked with Higher Stoke Risk
    http://www.americanheart.org/present.jhtml?indentifier=3008854

8.8 HYPERTENSION

Hypertension is regarded as one of the most important public health problems of today as well as a very common cardiovascular disease. It is preventable, easily detectable and treatable.

It not only is regarded as a key CVD in itself, but also, as a major risk factor for other CVDs such as carotid artery disease, cerebral artery disease/stroke, coronary artery disease and peripheral artery disease and their consequences, if left untreated.

As hypertension already has been reviewed previously, it will not be discussed further in this section. The reader is referred to Chapter 7—*Hypertension* for basic information on hypertension and references for additional information.

8.9 KIDNEY DISEASE

Chronic kidney disease (CKD) is a known, major modifiable risk factor for CVD and its incidence is on the rise. An estimated 4.5 percent of adults have clinical evidence of chronic kidney disease. The rate of kidney failure in the United States has doubled in the past decade. While many people with kidney disease will never develop kidney failure, others will, joining more than 400,000 people annually treated with dialysis or a kidney transplant. CVD now accounts for half of all deaths among people with kidney failure

Recent clinical studies now reinforce the importance of early detection of CKD not only to slow progression to kidney failure but also to identify it as a significant risk factor for CVD.

CKD may be defined by an estimated glomerular filtration rate (GFR) of less than 60 ml/min/1.73 m^2, a measure of how well the kidneys are filtering waste chemicals from blood.

The National Institute of Diabetes and Digestive and Kidney Disease (NIDDK) at the NIH followed more than 1 million adults from the Kaiser Permanente Renal Registry in San Francisco for nearly 3 years (average age 52) and found that when kidney function (glomerular filtration rate—GFR) fell significantly below normal, the risk of death as well as cardiovascular events such as heart disease, myocardial infarction and stroke, and hospitalization increased. Compared to patients whose GFR was at least 60 ml per minute per 1.73 m², the increased risk of:

- death ranged from 17 percent in those whose GFR was between 45 and 59, and increased to about 600 percent in those whose GFR was less than 15

- CVD events ranged from 43 percent in those whose GFR was between 45 and 59, and increased to 343 percent in those whose GFR was less than 15, and

- hospitalization ranged from 14 percent in those whose GFR was between 45 and 59, and increased to 315 percent in those whose GFR was less than 15

Regular serum creatinine testing and the MDRD equation have been used to estimate GFR in adults at high risk for kidney disease—those with diabetes, high blood pressure, or a family history of kidney problems, especially African Americans, Hispanic Americans and Native Americans.

Additional information on the kidney and CVD is available at:

- Medical Calculator
  GFR Estimation Using the MDRD Equation
  (Modification of Diet in Renal Disease Study Group)
  http://medcalc3000.com/GFREstimate.htm
- National Institute of Diabetes and Digestive and Kidney Diseases
  Kidney Disease Overview
  http://www.nkdep.nih.gov/patients
- New England Journal of Medicine

Chronic Kidney Disease and the Risk of Death, Cardiovascular Events, and Hospitalization, NEJM 2004; 351:1296-1305

Relation between Renal Dysfunction and Cardiovascular Outcomes After Myocardial Infarction, NEJM 2004; 351: 1285-1295

8.10 METABOLIC SYNDROME X

Metabolic syndrome x is a major modifiable risk factor for CVD.

Metabolic syndrome x is the simultaneous occurrence of multiple cardiovascular risk factors in an individual that approximately doubles the risk of coronary artery disease and stroke. This condition is also known as syndrome x, insulin resistance syndrome, and dysmetabolic syndrome.

A national health survey revealed that more than one in five Americans has the metabolic syndrome x. This syndrome increases in prevalence with age and is reported by the Centers for Disease Control and Prevention (CDC) to affect at least 45 to 50 million adults in the United States. These findings highlight the need to identify and treat these individuals as soon as possible in order to reduce the risk of CVD.

Researchers at the CDC/NIH, as part of ATP III (Third Report of the National Cholesterol Education Program Expert Panel for Detection, Evaluation, and Treatment of High Blood Cholesterol in Adults) indicates that a diagnosis of metabolic syndrome x is made when a person has three or more of the following:

- waistline of 40 inches (102 cm) for men, 35 inches (88 cm) for women
- blood pressure of 130/85 mmHg or higher

- triglyercide levels above 150 mg/dl
- fasting blood glucose level greater than 100–110 mg/dl
- High density lipoprotein <40 mg/dl in men, <50 mg/dl in women

Three groups of people are reported to be likely to develop metabolic syndrome x, namely:

- individuals with diabetes who have difficulty maintaining blood sugar levels in the normal range
- those without diabetes who have hyperinsulinemia (high blood insulin levels) without glucose intolerance and have hypertension
- heart attack survivors who have hyperinsulinemia without glucose intolerance

Usually metabolic syndrome x patients are asymptomatic. Consistently high blood levels of insulin and glucose may lead to type II diabetes mellitus and CVD.

Since physical inactivity and excess weight are the main underlying factors in the development of metabolic syndrome x, diet, exercise and weight control are key to preventing this disorder and complications associated with it. In addition, blood pressure and lipids need to be normalized, and a calorie restricted diet with carbohydrate intake at no more than 50 percent of total calories consumed. Foods eaten should include:

- those containing complex carbohydrates and unrefined sugars
- ones having high fiber content such as beans, whole grains, fruits and vegetables
- poultry and fish rather than "red" meats, and healthy fats such as canola oil, olive oil, flaxseed oil and nuts and seeds.

In addition, consumption of alcohol should be limited to one drink a day for women or two drinks for men.

Additional information on metabolic syndrome x is available at:
* American Heart Association
  Metabolic Syndrome X
  http://www.americanheart.org.presenter.jhtml?identifier=4756
* Cleveland Clinic Heart Center
  Deadly Quartet of Metabolic Risk Factors Increases Mortality CAD
  http://www.clevelandclinic.org/heartcenter/pub/professionals/cardio-consult/2001/spring/syndromex.htm

8.11 ORAL CONTRACEPTIVES

The risk for cardiovascular disease (CVD) is significantly lower with current preparations of low-dose contraceptives, including those that contain the new progestrogens, than with older contraceptives containing high doses of estrogen. Among users of low-dose oral contraceptives, CVD usually occurs in smokers and women with other predisposing risk factors. Every effort should be made to encourage smoking cessation among users of oral contraceptives in order to reduce CVD risk.

8.12 OVERWEIGHT/OBESITY

Overweight/obesity remains one of the major modifiable risk factors for CVD.

Large waist circumference (>40 inches in men and 35 in women) and a high waist-to-hip ratio are significant CVD risk factors in overweight/obese individuals.

Dyslipidemia (combinations of high blood total cholesterol and/or triglycerides), high LDL (low density lipoprotein cholesterol) and low HDL (high density lipoprotein cholesterol) further dispose individuals to the risk for CVD.

Over 50 percent of overweight/obese individuals suffer from hypertension (high blood pressure). Studies show a direct relationship between android or central obesity and hypertension, coronary artery disease, and stroke.

Carotid artery, cerebral artery, stroke and peripheral arterial disease also are not uncommon complications, especially in individuals with hypertension and a high waist-to-hip ratio.

Overweight/obese individuals often suffer from a disorder called metabolic syndrome x which puts them at high risk for coronary artery disease, stroke and type 2 diabetes mellitus.

Cardiomyopathy, fatty infiltration of the heart leading to heart failure, appears to be closely related to the duration of obesity. This complication is reported to occur more commonly in those individuals who have been obese for 10 or more years.

The death rate from CVD is reported to be around 50 percent higher for those who are moderately obese and 90 percent higher for those with severe obesity. Diet, exercise, weight loss, and lifestyle changes and certain medications significantly reduce the development of CVD in overweight/obese individuals.

In men, 50 percent or greater above normal weight, mortality rates are increased approximately two fold, five fold for diabetics and four fold in those with digestive tract disease. In females, with the same percentage weight gain over normal, mortality is increased two fold, in those with diabetes mortality is increased eight fold, and three fold in those with digestive tract disease. Overweight individuals of both sexes especially younger overweight individuals, tend to die significantly sooner than their lean contemporaries. Most cases of death in both sexes are primarily due to various forms of CVD.

Overweight/obesity are now considered to represent a serious threat to the health of the United States (and the developed countries) accounting for:
- 90–95 percent of all type 2 diabetes mellitus, itself a key risk factor for CVD
- 50–70 percent of all CVD
- 35 percent of all hypertension, a key risk factor for CVD

The degree of overweight/obesity and body fat content are estimated clinically by measuring body mass index (BMI), waist and hip circumferences and their ratio, and skin-fold thickness in selected areas. All of these methods together provide a reasonably good estimate of overweight, obesity, and body fat content and distribution.

An expert panel convened by the National Institute of Health has recommended that Body Mass Index (BMI) be used to classify overweight and obesity. This was done because BMI:

- correlates well with total body fat for the majority of people as well as with the risk of complications and death (e.g. heart disease increases with BMI in all population groups)
- calculation is simple, rapid and inexpensive with a calculator—also using a table/normogram

BMI is a measure of weight in relation to height determined by the formula:

BMI = weight in pounds divided by height in inches squared times 703

A BMI calculator is available at:

- Center for Disease Control and Prevention
  BMI—Body Mass Index: BMI Calculator
  http://www.cdc.gov/nccdphp/dnpa/bmi/calc-bmi.htm

A table to estimate BMI is available at:

- National Heart, Lung and Blood Institute
  Body Mass Index Table
  http://www.nhlbi.nih.gov/guidelines/obesity/bmi_tbl.htm

Classification of BMI and corresponding medical risk is given in the table below.

Overweight/Obesity and CVD Risk

Classification	BMI	CVD Risk
Healthy weight	18.5–24.9	very low risk
Overweight	25.0–29.9	low risk
Obesity		
Mild, Class I	30.0–34.9	moderate risk
Moderate, Class II	35.0–39.9	high risk
Severe, Class III	>40.0	very high risk

Two basic fat distribution patterns exist in overweight and obese persons. One is called android (apple-shaped or central, chiefly around the abdomen). The other is designated as gynoid (pear-shaped or gluteofemoral, principally around the hips, buttocks, and thighs). These two types can be differentiated visually or classified by the ratio of waist-to-hip circumference. The presence of excess body fat around the abdomen, when out of proportion to total body fat, is considered an independent risk factor for CVD.

Waist circumference is a common measure used to assess abdominal fat content. A waist circumference over 40 inches (102 centimeters) for men and 35 inches for women (88 centimeters) is considered to be android or central obesity, and is more closely correlated with CVD and death. Hip circumference greater than waist is called gynoid or gluteofemoral obesity. waist-to-hip ratio of less than 0.8 in women and less than 1.0 in men are considered normal.

All overweight/obese individual should aim for a healthy weight. The NIH Expert Panel on Identification, Evaluation and Treatment of Overweight and Obesity in Adults recommends weight loss in overweight/obese individuals in order to:

- lower elevated blood pressure in those with hypertension
- decrease levels of total cholesterol, LDL cholesterol, and triglycerides and raise low levels of HDL cholesterol in those with dyslipidemia
- normalize blood glucose and insulin levels in those with diabetes mellitus
- reduce body weight by at least 10 percent from initial baseline, and, if successful, further weight loss can be attempted until normal weight is achieved. Weight loss should be targeted at 1–2 pounds per week for a period up to 6 months with subsequent strategy based on the total amount of weight lost.

A calorie restricted, low to moderate fat diet should be considered in treatment. Reducing fat intake as part of the low calorie diet is a practical way to reduce calories in the diet.

Physical activity (PA) should be used as part of a comprehensive weight loss/weight control program. PA modestly contributes to weight loss and may help to decrease abdominal fat and increase cardio-respiratory fitness. All adults who are capable should set a long-term goal to accumulate at least 30–60 (preferably 60) minutes of moderate-intensity physical activity/exercise on most, if not all, days of the week.

Additional information is available at:

- National Institute of Diabetes, Digestive and Kidney Diseases
  Do You Know the Health Risks of Being Overweight/Obese?
  http://www.niddk.nih.gov/health/nurit/pubs/health.htm

- National Heart Lung and Blood Institute
  Clinical Guidelines on the Identification, Evaluation and Treatment of Overweight and Obesity in Adults
  http://www.nhlbi.nih.gov/guidelines/obesity/sum_evid.htm
  Practical Guide to the Identification, Evaluation and Treatment of Overweight and Obesity in Adults
  http://www.nhlbi.nih.gov/guidelines/obesity/pretgd_c.pdf

8.13 OXIDATIVE STRESS/ANTIOXIDANTS

Introduction

Oxidative stress occurs when the production of reactive oxygen species (ROS) exceeds the capacity of the body's antioxidant defense mechanisms to neutralize or detoxify them, leading to oxidative damage to macromolecules and cells. Oxidants may be formed by many metabolic and environmental processes. They also are released by phagocytes, neutrophils, and macrophages during their role in early immune defenses against pathogens. However, in chronic inflammation ROS may result in host tissue damage and pathology.

Serious consequences for cells due to oxidative damage may occur as a result of three basic factors, namely:
- an increase in oxidant generation
- decrease in antioxidant protection
- failure of the body to repair oxidative damage

Oxidative stress-mediated cell damage occurs via reactive oxygen species (ROS) produced continually in most tissues and this is regarded as part of normal cell function. However, ROS generation may increase significantly in atherosclerosis and CVD.

ROS include such molecules as hydrogen peroxide, ions like hypochlorite, radicals like the hydroxyl radical and the superoxide ion which is both ion and radical. Radicals, also called "free radicals", contain an unpaired electron in their outermost orbit of electrons resulting in an unstable configuration. As a result, radicals quickly react with other molecules to achieve a more stable state.

In the arterial vascular system, formation of ROS from endothelial and smooth muscle cells and macrophages seem to be of major relevance regarding the atherosclerotic process due in a large part to a reaction with nitric oxide resulting in:

- attenuation of endothelium-dependent dilation leading to disturbed organ perfusion and systemic hypertension
- induction of cellular damage and inflammation
- apoptosis (cell death)
- interference with intracellular signaling processes

The main source of ROS is aerobic cellular respiration taking place in the mitochondria. Under normal conditions ROS are cleared from the cell by such enzymatic systems as superoxide dismutases (SODs), catalase, and glutathione, and uric acid. These substances, along with others, are important for protecting the cardiovascular system from oxidative stress damage. For example, low levels of serum glutathione in adolescent boys has been cited as an independent predictor of parental coronary artery disease

Oxidative stress has been identified throughout the process of atherosclerosis, beginning at the earliest stages of endothelial dysfunction. As the process of atherosclerosis proceeds, inflammatory cells, as well as other constituents of atherosclerotic plaques release large amounts of ROS which, in turn, facilitates further atherogenesis.

Hyperlipidemia is considered a major inducer of oxidative stress and plays a pivotal role in atherogenesis. In the atherosclerotic process, ROS oxidizes lipids and resultant oxidatively modified LDL (ox-LDL) becomes a much more potent proatherosclerotic mediator. Statins (HMG-CoA reductase inhibitors) have been shown to reduce susceptibility of LDL to oxidation by ROS. This provides evidence supporting an antioxidant effect of statin drugs, as an important action independent of their lipid lowering effect.

Hypertension and hyperlipidemia are major risk factors for CVD (e.g coronary artery disease) and both are often present in the same patient. Common effects of hyperlipidemia and hypertension in the atherosclerotic process include the fact that both:

- stimulate ROS production
- degrade or decrease endothelial nitric oxide synthase and decrease endothelium-dependent vasodilation
- are pro-inflammatory states favoring adhesion of molecules and clotting
- cause apoptosis (cell death)
- activate signal transduction pathways.

All this may lead to such diseases as atherosclerosis, carotid artery disease, coronary artery disease, cerebral artery disease/stroke and peripheral artery disease.

Inhibition of ROS generation and function serves as a potential therapy to attenuate the extent and severity of atherosclerosis and its consequences. Major risk factors involved in atherosclerosis stimulate ROS generation and interdependently induce atherogenesis. Concurrent therapy directed at modification of major risk factors may block oxidative stress and resultant atherogenesis and its complications.

Oxidative Stress and Diabetes Mellitus

Researchers have found that oxidative stress plays a role in the damage to tissues caused by diabetes mellitus, itself an important CVD risk factor. Japanese scientists have demonstrated that oxidative stress damages the insulin-producing cells of the pancreas in rats which can worsen diabetes, and antioxidant supplements in animals may reduce that damage. There is growing evidence that excess generation of highly reactive free radicals, largely due to hyperglycemia, causes oxidative stress in humans, which further exacerbates the development and progression of diabetes and its complications. However, despite a great deal of evidence on oxidative stress and its role in experimental diabetes in animals, large scale clinical trials with classic antioxidants have failed to demonstrate significant benefit for diabetic patients to date.

Oxidative Stress and Smoking

Cigarette smoke contains large amount of free radicals which may lead to an increased oxidative stress state in smokers. Psychological stress itself also can cause oxidative stress and a heightened proinflammatory/prooxidant state. And smokers generally have higher psychological stress levels which is thought to explain, in part at least, why they smoke so much. Thus, smoking is an important cause of oxidative stress and this may help explain why cigarette smoking is such an important CVD risk factor.

Oxidative Stress and Kidney Disease

Patients affected by end-stage renal disease (ESRD) experience an excess morbidity and mortality due to cardiovascular disease which cannot be fully explained by the classical CVD risk factors. Among emerging CVD risk factors, oxidative stress is currently being given emphasis since it may be implicated in the pathogenesis of atherosclerosis and other complications of ESRD. However, further controlled clinical trials with anti-oxidants are required to establish evidence-based recommendations for clinical practice.

Oxidative Stress and Antioxidants

Since ROS are widely regarded to be involved in the initiation and progression of atherosclerosis, it is not surprising that antioxidant therapies constitute one of the most new and promising strategies available against this disease process. To date there are at least six classes of anti-atherogenic agents that have exhibited beneficial antioxidant effects to varying degrees. These are: 1) probucol, 2) statins such as simvastatin, 3) angiotension blockers, and ACE (angiotension converting enzyme) inhibitors such as enalapril, 4) vitamins E and C, etc., 5) certain lignands such as rosiglitazone and proglitazone, widely used to treat type II diabetes mellitus and 6) various food phytonutrients being evaluated for their therapeutic antioxidant effects. Newer agents are under development and one or more may become available in coming years.

Antioxidants and CVD

Elevated blood cholesterol, particularly the cholesterol carried by low density lipoprotein (LDL or "bad" cholesterol) is a major risk factor for CVD. Normally LDL in blood plasma is not oxidized and oxidation of LDL to any significant extent is regarded as a contributor to the development of atherosclerosis. Macrophage "scavenger" cells are reported to preferentially take up oxidized LDL, become over loaded with blood lipids, and convert into what is known as foam cells which then become part of the so called fatty streaks or plaques in the arteries, an early sign of atherosclerosis.

Humans produce auto-antibodies against oxidized LDL, and levels of such antibodies are found to be higher in patients with significant atherosclerosis.

The identification of LDL oxidation as a key event in atherosclerosis suggests that it may be possible to prevent it through diet modification or antioxidant supplementation. Epidemiological and other clinical data already strongly suggest that dietary antioxidants protect against CVD. However, to date, prospective clinical trials with antioxidant supplements have provided results which are considered equivocal at best. Nevertheless, this does not mean that antioxidants supplements do not work, rather it may means that much more research needs to be done to establish the use of antioxidant supplements in the prevention/treatment of CVD.

Additional information on oxidative stress/antioxidants is available at:

- American Heart Association
  Get Antioxidants from Food, Not Supplements
  http://www.americanheart.org/presenter.jhtml?identifier=3023709
- Indian Heart Journal
  Role of Oxidative Stress in Coronary Heart Disease by Chen, J. and Mehta, JL, Indian Heart Journal, March-April 2004, Vol. 5, pp. 1–18
  http://www.indianheartjournal.com/MarchApril2004/Role%20of/%20Oxidative%20Stress%20i
- National Heart Lung and Blood Institute
  Oxidative Stress/Inflammation and the Heart
  http://www.nhlbi.nih.gov
- Nutrition Institute of America
  Comprehensive Nutrient Review
  http://www.nutritioninstituteofamerica.org/research/NutrientReview/CodexIntrol.htm

8.14 PERIODONTAL DISEASE

Periodontal disease is a major modifiable risk factor for CVD. The word periodontal means "around the tooth". According to the American Academy of Periodontology, periodontal (gum) diseases, including gingivitis and periodontitis, are considered to be important dental infections which if left untreated, can lead to CVD.

Periodontitis is a chronic bacterial infection that affects the gums and bone supporting the teeth. It can affect one or many teeth and begins when the bacteria in plaque (the sticky, colorless film that constantly forms on your teeth) causes the gums to become infected. In the mildest form of the disease, gingivitis, the gums redden, swell and bleed easily. Gingivitis is often caused by inadequate oral hygiene and/or poor nutrition, and is reversible with professional treatment and good oral hygiene/care. Untreated gingivitis can advance to periodontitis. With time, plaque can spread and grow below the gum line. Toxins produced by the bacteria in plaque irritate the gums and stimulate a chronic inflammatory response in which the body, in essence, turns on itself and the tissues and bone that support the teeth decay and are eventually destroyed. Gums separate from the teeth, forming pockets (spaces between the teeth and gums), and subsequently more gum and bone tissues are destroyed. Often, this destructive inflammatory process can lead to teeth that develop caries, and become loose and may have to be removed.

Diseased gums release significantly higher levels of bacterial pro-inflammatory components such as endotoxins into the blood stream in patients with periodontal disease and may trigger the liver to make C-reactive protein (CRP), a predictor for increased risk for CVD. Approximately15 percent of adults between 21 and 50 years old, and 30 percent of adults over 50 are reported to have periodontal disease representing a major modifiable risk factor when associated with elevations of CRP in blood.

Researchers have known for quite some time that elevated CRP levels increase the risk for CVD. A more recent study published in the New England Journal of Medicine identified elevated CRP levels as a stronger predictor of heart attacks than elevated cholesterol levels, and recommended both CRP and cholesterol screening for more accurate risk assessment for CVD.

Thus, it is important to treat and eliminate any existing periodontal disease in order to reduce risk for CVD.

Additional information on periodontal disease is available at:
*   American Academy of Periodontology
    Periodontal Diseases
    http://www.perio.org/consumer/2a.html
    Periodontal Disease, C-Reactive Protein and Overall Health
    http://www.perio.org/consumer/happy-heart.htm
    New Study Confirms Periodontal Disease Linked to Heart Disease
    http://www.perio.org/consumer/bacteria.htm

8.15 PSYCHOLOGICAL STRESS

Stress is considered a major modifiable risk factor for CVD. Although stress is not considered to be a traditional risk factor by some, researchers have noted an important relationship between CVD and stress. In the prevention and/or treatment of CVD, stress needs to be minimized and controlled in so far as possible.

Stress may be regarded as the psychological and physiological response produced by internal and/or external forces calling on an individual to adapt, thus undergoing a stress response. This may occur as the result of either pleasant or unpleasant experiences or forces called stressors. Such things as anxiety, ecstasy, depression, sorrow, joy, sexual arousal, worry, pain, trauma, disease, death in the family or of a close friend, occupational factors, relationship/family problems, or excessive heat or cold, etc. all may induce the psychological and physiological manifestations/consequences of stress. Consequently, stress is difficult and almost impossible to avoid.

Often individuals seek out stress in the form of adventure, excitement, thrills, and challenge for the joy it brings them. This has led to such pleasant stress as being referred to as eustress in contrast to the more troublesome and even malignant form of unpleasant emotional stress, known as distress. It is the intensity and duration of unpleasant stress (emotional distress), and consequent anxiety and/or depression resulting from it, along with the subsequent wear and tear on the body, that is of prime concern for the development of CVD.

Responses to Stress

A considerable body of evidence now indicates that the central nervous system plays a key role in the physiologic response to psychological stress (emotional distress). For example, an abundance of evidence exists regarding the occurrence of cardiac arrhythmias and even sudden death during emotionally distressful life events. And animal studies indicate that emotional stress can increase cardiac vulnerability to cardiac arrhythmias by as much as 50 percent.

Interestingly, psychological stress (emotional distress) and the anxiety/ depression produced by it are linked to all the traditional CVD risk factors in one way or another.

For example, serum cholesterol/triglycerides may be elevated by emotional stress and the anxiety/depression produced—total cholesterol and LDL rise, and HDL falls. In addition, it has been shown that relaxation techniques not only reduce stress but also the lipid changes associated with it.

Cigarette smoking also is stress-linked. The decision to smoke often is related to stress/anxiety/depression produced by life events. And, individuals who stop smoking "permanently" seem to develop better coping skills for dealing with stress.

Diabetic blood sugar levels, weight or caloric intake also can easily be negatively affected by stress and the anxiety and/or depression produced. This may be due, at least in part, to increased glucocorticoid and catecholamine release from the adrenals.

Stressed individuals also frequently overeat for "comfort", using "food as a tranquilizer". Therefore, overweight/obesity may be due to a stressful lifestyle and the anxiety/depression produced. Excessive food consumption and alcohol often are used by emotionally stressed individuals to reduce stress levels.

Stress/anxiety

A large number of studies also now support the view that stress/anxiety:
- are involved in the pathogenesis of hypertension
- can contribute to increased alcohol and food intake
- increases clotting factors in blood making it more likely that a clot will form leading to a stroke or heart attack.

Stressful situations may raise the heart rate and blood pressure, increasing the heart's need for oxygen. This can bring on angina pectoris and/or myocardial infarction in susceptible individuals with CAD.

During times of stress, the nervous system releases extra hormones which can injure the arteries, especially the arterial linings (endothelium), causing the walls to "thicken" and "harden", and for plaque to buildup on the inner wall stimulating the atherosclerotic process. Thus, individuals who have significant emotional distress, and unhealthy responses to such stress in their lives, have a greater risk for CVD.

Emotional stress can:
- make one feel angry, afraid, helpless or hopeless
- cause sleep disturbances and difficulties in going to sleep, staying asleep, and having a restful sleep
- give rise to aches or discomfort or pain in the head, neck, jaw and back
- lead to smoking, overeating, and drug abuse as well as anxiety and/or depression
- be so subtle that one may not even feel stressed even though the cardiovascular system may be suffering from it greatly

Remember that it is often very difficult to control outside forces/events in life that are stressful. However, one can change the perception of events and reduce stress effects on the cardiovascular system.

Persons who react to stress with anger, are reported to have three times the normal risk of developing CVD. Also, having a phobia or an extreme dislike increases one's likelihood of developing early fatal heart disease. In contrast having a positive attitude is reported to be one of the best overall means of reducing stress and preventing heart disease.

Stress/depression

Depression due to stress is a major, modifiable risk factor for heart disease along with other traditional ones. Much clinical research over the past two decades, has shown that depression and heart disease are common companions, and one can easily lead to the other. In fact, it has been said that "depression can break your heart".

Individuals who have a history of depression are reported to be four times more likely to suffer a heart attack in the next 10–14 years. In addition, heart attack patients who are depressed, are regarded as four times as likely to die in the next 6 months compared to those who are not depressed. Depression may:

- make it harder to take medications needed and to carry out necessary treatment for heart disease
- result in chronically elevated stress hormones such as cortisol and adrenaline, and the activation of the sympathetic nervous system, which can have deleterious effects on the heart and blood vessels.

People with heart disease are more likely to suffer from depression than otherwise healthy individuals. While around 1 in 20 American adults experience major depression in a given year, about 1 in 3 adults who have survived a heart attack become depressed. And, unfortunately most heart patients with depression do not receive appropriate treatment as both cardiologists and primary care physicians often overlook depression, or do not treat it adequately.

As the combination of depression and heart disease is associated with increased CVD and death, effective treatment of depression is imperative. Pharmacological and cognitive behavioral therapy treatments for depression and counseling are reasonably well-developed and play an important role in reducing the negative impact of depression. Exercise is also effective in reducing both depression and CVD. A recent study has demonstrated that an effective exercise program may be considered comparable to treatment with an antidepressant medication in terms of improving depressive symptoms in adults diagnosed with major depression. And, exercise is a major protective factor against CVD as well.

Additional information on depression and heart disease is available at:

*   National Institute of Mental Health
    Depression and Heart Disease
    http://www.nimh.nih.gov/publicat/depheart.cfm

Stress management

Because of its importance, stress management has not only become a major part of the prevention but also the treatment of CVD. Some tips for preventing and/or controlling stress include the following:

*   mediate, engage in mindfulness
*   take note of things that cause you to feel stressed
*   try not to worry and concern yourself about outside things you can't control like someone else's behavior, another's belief systems, the weather, etc.

- prepare for upcoming events you know may be stressful, like a medical exam, job interview, or a move to a new location
- regard change as a positive challenge, not a threat
- work to peacefully resolve family, job and other conflicts
- seek friends, family members, or professional figures for help when needed
- establish realistic goals in life at home, and at work
- take control of your schedule and prioritize what needs to be done each day
- engage in physical activity and exercise on a regular basis
- eat well-balanced, nutritious meals and obtain enough restful sleep
- enjoy sports, social events, hobbies and other interesting activities
- give stress a holiday—go on a vacation and take time to enjoy life doing the things you like to do
- find your purpose in life, follow your bliss and live a healthy lifestyle

There are many forms of meditation. Choose one to your liking. Meditation is a simple natural technique to be practiced once or twice a day for 20–30 minutes each time. It is claimed that individuals who practice meditation live longer compared with those who don't, and may experience up to a 25 percent reduction in death from all causes. Studies indicate that meditation may effectively reduce stress, lower blood pressure, and prevent CVD.

While emotional problems of every day living can be upsetting, and one may feel stressed as a result, it is important to remember that it is not the outside stressors/forces that are of primary concern but rather the perception and reaction to such. In this regard, the basic message of the "serenity prayer" teaches an effective way for reducing stress, namely learn to:

- change the things that can be changed
- accept the things that cannot be changed
- have the wisdom to know the difference between the two

Additional information on stress is available at:
- American Academy of Family Practice
  Stress: How to Cope with Life's Challenge
  http://familydoctor.org/167.xml?printx
- Cleveland Clinic
  Stress Management and Your Heart
  http://www.clevelandclinic.org/heartcenter/pub/guide/prevention/
  stress/stressheart.htm
- Mind/Body Medical Institute
  Harvard Medical School/Beth Israel-Deaconess Medical Center
  Managing Stress/Mindfulness
  http://www.mbmi.org
- UCLA School of Medicine
  Stress Management
  http://www.womenshealth.med.ucla.edu/patients/stress.htm

8.16 SEDENTARY LIFESTYLE

Sedentary lifestyle is not only a major risk factor for CVD but also one of the ten leading causes of chronic disease, disability and death in the world. Physical inactivity increases all causes of mortality and doubles the risk of CVD, type II diabetes and obesity. It significantly increases the risk of hypertension as well.

Levels of inactivity are high in virtually all developed countries including the United States. In the rapidly growing cities, especially the larger ones, physical inactivity is an even greater problem. Crowding, poverty, crime, traffic, lack of parks/sports and recreation facilities, and sidewalks make physical activity difficult.

Even in rural areas, sedentary pastimes, such as watching television have become increasingly popular. Inevitably, the results are increased levels of obesity, diabetes, and CVD. Unhealthy diets, excessive caloric intake, inactivity and obesity leading to CVD and other chronic diseases have become the greatest public health problem in most countries in the developed world, including the United States.

Data gathered from health surveys around the world is remarkably consistent—the proportion of adults who are sedentary, or nearly so, ranges from 60 to 85 percent. In the United States, only approximately 20 percent or so of US adults participate in regular, sustained physical activity during leisure-time. And the prevalence of regular, vigorous physical activity in the US is reported to be only around 15 percent or so of those over age 18.

Americans are just not getting enough physical activity/exercise. The reason for this is that lives in the US are complex/multifaceted and stressed, and may also include the fact that many Americans are exercising for the wrong reason(s).

Of the individuals who believe that physical activity/exercise is important, many believe the overwhelming reasons to incorporate activity/exercise into one's life is to change the outward appearance of the body. Rather, the emphasis should center around the many physical, psychological, and health benefits and de-emphasizing just the changing of outward appearance. When weight loss becomes a primary goal, one may become discouraged when failing to lose desired pounds or regaining lost weight.

In combination with caloric restriction, moderate-intensity daily physical activity/exercise:

- burns calories, and increases the caloric deficit and weight loss (physical activity/exercise alone without caloric restriction usually produces only modest weight loss)
- improves lean body mass and minimizes muscle loss
- reduces feelings of anxiety, depression and stress, and elevates mood and the feeling of well-being
- improves general fitness, mobility, and the ability to perform activities of daily living
- facilitates cardiovascular and muscular fitness
- decreases insulin resistance and type 2 diabetes mellitus
- reduces elevated blood cholesterol and body fat
- lowers the risk of CVD

Many of the benefits of physical activity/exercise occur even if weight loss is not very great (e.g., up to 10 percent) and even if one remains overweight or obese. In any event, it is important to remember that there is a significant decrease in CVD and overall mortality rate in those who are physically active and exercise compared to those who remain sedentary.

It is generally recommended that one engage in 30–60 (preferably 60) minutes of moderate intensity physical activity/exercise daily, 5–7 (preferably 7) days, a week.

To be successful, a physical activity/exercise program needs to be done at a safe comfort level and easily fit into the daily living routine. Preferably it should be done under a physician's supervision. One should start out slowly and gradually increase activity/exercise to moderate-intensity over the course of a few weeks time. Trying too hard at first may lead to injury and prove to be counterproductive.

To reduce the risk of CVD, one needs to leave the sedentary lifestyle behind and live a physically active life which includes a significant level of daily exercise.

Additional information is available at:
- National Heart Lung and Blood Institute
  Guide to Physical Activity
  http://www.nhlbi.nih.gov/health/public/heart/obesity/lose_wt/phy_act.htm
- Just Move.Org
  How to Implement Physical Activity in Primary and Secondary Prevention: Benefits of Daily Physical Activity
  http://www.justmove.org/fitnessnews/health.cfm?target=dailybene.html
- World Health Organization
  Sedentary Lifestyle: A Global Public Health Problem
  http://www.who.int

8.17 Smoking/Secondhand Smoke

Smoking

Smoking is a major risk factor and one of the most preventable, modifiable risk factors for CVD and stroke. It acts along with other risk factors to greatly increase the risk for coronary artery disease (CAD) and other CVDs. Even one to two cigarettes a day increases the risk for CVD.

Cigarette smoking also remains a major independent risk factor for sudden cardiac death in patients with coronary artery disease. In this regard, smokers have around twice the risk of nonsmokers.

People who smoke cigars or pipes seem to have a higher risk of death from CAD and stroke but their risk for the development of CVD in general is not considered as great as for cigarette smokers.

According to the American Heart Association, more than 400,000 Americans die each year from smoking related diseases and many of these deaths are due to the effects of smoking on the heart and arteries in the body. Research has shown that smoking increases heart rate, causes constriction of the arteries, and creates irregular heartbeats, all of which make the heart and the arteries work harder. Smoking also raises blood pressure which increases the risk of a heart attack and stroke in people who already have high blood pressure. Nicotine, tar, and carbon monoxide in smoke also are harmful. These chemicals and others lead to oxidative stress, the buildup of fatty plaques in the arteries, and hardening of the arteries (atherosclerosis) restricting the normal flow of blood. Along with increased levels of fibrinogen caused by smoking this can lead to clotting and a heart attack or stroke.

In order to significantly reduce the risk of CVD, one must quit smoking. In the first year after stopping smoking, risk of CAD and other CVD drops sharply and returns to "normal" over time.

Only around one third of smokers attempt to stop smoking each year and around one in five seek professional help for smoking cessation. And, less than 10 percent of smokers who attempt to quit on their own are successful over the long term. A number of clinical trials have demonstrated that both drug treatment and professional counseling are effective in bringing about more lasting smoking cessation. While each of these two approaches is effective alone, the two combined are reported to achieve the highest rates of smoking cessation. Physician counseling is reported to double the cessation rate compared with no intervention, and is regarded as more effective compared with just advising the patient to quit.

Six products are now approved for smoking cessation by the Food and Drug Administration. These are buproion and five nicotine replacement medications (gum, lozenge, transdermal patch, nasal spray and a vapor inhaler). These products each are reported to increase the long term rates of smoking cessation.

If you don't smoke, don't start.

Secondhand Smoke

New studies suggest that even small amounts of secondhand smoke can cause life-threatening changes to a nonsmoker's circulatory system. While the immediate effects of secondhand exposure to smoke are reversed within a few hours, exposure to secondhand smoke over longer periods of time can have significant consequences for the heart, including an increased risk for coronary artery disease and an acute coronary event such as a heart attack or long-term development of atherosclerosis.

Chronic exposure to secondhand smoke is reported to be about 80 percent as deleterious to health as being a pack-a-day smoker. The cardiovascular system is exquisitely sensitive to the toxins of secondhand cigarette smoke. And, most of the toxic effects of secondhand smoke occur as early as the first few minutes of exposure.

Dr. Stanton A. Glantz, Professor of Medicine and longtime antismoking advocate at the University of California, San Francisco and his colleague, Dr. Joaquin Barnoya, an Assistant Adjunct Professor of Epidemiology at UCSF reviewed the existing medical literature on the effect of secondhand smoke on the cardiovascular system and reported their finding in the May 24, 2004 issue of *Circulation*. They reviewed 29 studies published since 1995 that compared the effects of secondhand smoke with the effects of active smoking and found that:

- there is sufficient evidence that key aspects of cardiovascular function, including clotting, ability of blood vessels to change size, arterial stiffness, atherosclerosis, oxidative stress, inflammation, heart rate variability, energy metabolism, and severity of heart attack are all sensitive to the toxins found in secondhand smoke

- effects of even brief (minutes to hours) of exposure to passive smoking (secondhand smoke) are often nearly as large (averaging around 80–90 percent) as chronic active smoking.

These authors have argued that it doesn't take much secondhand smoke to cause big adverse cardiovascular effects. Therefore, if one already has compromised coronary circulation and goes into a smoky environment, there is a substantial increase in risk for an acute event such as a heart attack. They also point out that non-smokers are more sensitive to the effects of tobacco smoke than are active smokers, and in some cases, the effects of secondhand smoke are as large or even larger than one sees in an active smoker.

Secondhand smoke injures, disables and kills people by virtue of its cardiovascular effects, and also by its effects on the lung. Society should not permit tobacco smoke to be imposed secondhand on others. Smoking in public places needs to be banned—not just by some states but by all-and this needs to be done sooner rather than later.

Accordingly, the dangers appear to be so great that all of us should avoid secondhand smoke as much as possible and fight for smoke-free workplaces and public places, fully supporting cessation of smoking campaigns/programs everywhere.

Additional information on smoking/secondhand smoke is available at:
- American Heart Association
  Risk Factors for Coronary Heart Diseases
  http://www.americanheart.org/presenter.jhtml?identifier=4726

Smoking is a Women's Single Biggest Risk Factor

http://www.americanheart.org/presenter.jhtml?identifier=2779

Smoking Cessation

http://www.americanheart.org/presenter.jhtml?identifier=4731

- Penn State Heart and Vascular Institute

  Risk Factors for Cardiovascular Disease

  http://www.hmc.psu.edu/heartandvascular/patient/articles/pe099.htm

- Cleveland Clinic Heart Center

  Preventing and Reversing Cardiovascular Disease

  http://www.clevelandclinic.org/heartcenter/pub/guide/prevention/riskfactors.htm

- Texas Heart Institute

  Heart Disease Risk Factors

  http://www.texasheartinstitute.org/riskfact.html

- US Food and Drug Administration

  Risk Factors for Cardiovascular Disease

  http://www.fda.gov/hearthealth/riskfactors/riskfactors/html

CHAPTER 9

▼

PREVENTION GUIDELINES FOR CVD

9.1 PREVENTION IS THE MAIN GOAL

Prevention is the main goal because once developed, CVD is difficult to reverse.

Most individuals do not pay close enough attention to their health or become aware of the possibility of developing CVD. Rather, they tend to deny the possibility by not recognizing that:

- a family history of premature CVD is important in determining risk in their own life
- their unhealthy lifestyle is a major factor in the risk for CVD
- the development of CVD is a gradual, lifelong process that cannot be seen or felt in the early stages
- prevention is the best option for avoiding CVD and its consequences
- there is a need to take charge, control and responsibility for their own cardiovascular health and do something about it "before it is too late"

CVD occurs with increasing frequency with advancing age and has become a leading cause of chronic disease, disability and death. Now that people are living longer, more productive lives than ever before because of the many advances in medicine, nutrition, new drugs, and other technology, it is more important than ever for individuals to act to prevent CVD as one of the main goals of their adult life.

9.2 ADOPT A HEALTHY LIFESTYLE

A key factor in the successful prevention of CVD lies in the adoption of a healthy lifestyle.

A healthy lifestyle refers to personal "good" behavior and habits such as:
- know/control modifiable risk factors for CVD disease
- exercise daily/avoid sedentary lifestyle
- eat sensibly/nutritious foods
- control/normalize blood pressure
- control/normalize blood lipids
- prevent/manage diabetes
- stop smoking/avoid secondhand smoke
- reduce/cope with stress

Adopting a healthy lifestyle and taking steps to prevent CVD should begin as early as possible in one's life and no later than around mid life, before age 40–45.

Additional information on healthy lifestyle is available at:
- Agency for Healthcare Research and Quality
  The Pocket Guide to Good Health for Adults
  http://www.ahrq.gov/ppip/adguide/adquide/pdf

- American Academy of Family Practice
  Healthy Living: What You Can Do To Keep Your Health
  http://familydoctor.org/0.86.xml
- Healthy People 2010
  http://www.healthypeople.gov/BeHealthy
  http://www.healthypeople.gov/LHI/Priorities.htm
  http://www.healthypeople.gov/LHI/Resources.htm
- National Institute of Health
  Healthy Lifestyles
  http://www.health.nih.gov

9.3 KNOW/MODIFY YOUR CVD PROFILE

Taking charge, control, and responsibility means, among other things that one needs to:

- know what CVD risk factors are all about
- "own" those risk factors that apply to oneself, and
- do something meaningful about the ones that are controllable/modifiable

In this way, risk can be minimized, and CVD prevented. However, one could do "all the right things" and still develop CVD because so may factors appear to be involved, some of which are known and controllable, and others are not. Nevertheless, by modifying known risk factors as well as is possible, it is likely that CVD may be successfully prevented in many cases, or at least delayed in its appearance for years.

As the CVD process may begin early in life and be silent, the presence or absence of risk factors should be assessed by mid-life—or even at a younger age if circumstances warrant. In deciding when to do so, it should be kept in mind that men generally are at increased CVD risk at age 45 and older whereas women usually are so at age 60–65 and older.

A basic assessment may include such things as:

- a complete history and physical exam
- battery of laboratory tests plus special procedures as indicated, and
- other evaluations deemed appropriate by the physician conducting the evaluation/assessment

Modifiable risk factors found should be treated and the patient should be followed up on an appropriate schedule established by their healthcare provider/physician.

In cases where no modifiable CVD risk factors are found in the initial assessment, a follow-up evaluation may be considered about every 5 years depending on circumstances.

9.4 ENGAGE IN PHYSICAL ACTIVITY/EXERCISE

Physical activity/exercise is essential for controlling certain risk factors and preventing CVD.

Engage in physical activity/exercise, 30–60 (preferably 60) minutes a day 5–7 (preferably 7) days a week. In one's daily activities, just keep moving as much as possible and avoid the sedentary lifestyle.

Daily aerobic exercise lowers blood pressure and improves blood lipid levels and helps to achieve and maintain normal weight, control blood sugar levels/diabetes, and reduce stress. Brisk walking and/or aerobics are regarded as excellent forms of exercise. The best exercise program is one that feels good and can be done over and over again without fail—hopefully for the rest of one's life.

Additional information on the health benefits of physical activity are available at:

- Just Move.org
  Benefits of Daily Physical Activity
  http://www.justmove.org/fitness/health/cfm?target=dailybene.html
- National Center for Chronic Disease Prevention and Health Promotion
  Physical Activity for Everyone: the Importance of Physical Activity
  http://www.cdc.gov/nccdphp.dnpa/physical/importance/index.htm

9.5 EAT SENSIBLY/NUTRITIOUS FOODS

If one expects to prevent CVD, it makes sense to eat a healthy CVD preventive diet. This means following the principles laid down by the American Heart Association and Dietary Guidelines for Americans which provide for:

- balanced levels of caloric intake and physical activity/exercise to achieve and maintain a normal weight, fitness, and good health
- a nutritionally balanced diet including 5–9 servings (preferably 9) of fruits, and vegetables daily, and one high in fiber
- at least a few servings daily of a variety of grains, principally whole grains
- limited intake of food high in saturated fat, trans fats, cholesterol, and sugar
- at least two servings of fish per week
- no more than 2.4 grams of sodium (6 grams of sodium chloride—salt) daily

- adequate potassium daily (around 4 grams or more)
- no more than 1–2 ounces of alcohol per day (1–2 drinks in men and 1 in women)

Limiting intake of trans fats in the diet is now considered to be even more important than saturated fats. Therefore, trans fats should be reduced as much as possible in any CVD preventive diet. The Institute of Medicine has concluded that there is no safe level of trans fats in the diet, and no sound reason to continue to consume them. Read the food labels and minimize intake of trans fat.

Adequate fluid intake averaging around 1.5–2.0 liters daily also is important. However, drinking soft water is not a good idea as it appears to be a definite risk factor for CVD. It lacks the minerals calcium and magnesium and replaces them with sodium which has a tendency to raise blood pressure and worsen the atherosclerotic process. And, magnesium deficiency in the diet is now recognized as a CVD risk factor. In addition, it is known that areas of the United States where people drink soft water have more CVD and heart attacks. Thus it is best to drink unsoftened water, or spring or well water.

Finally, there is increasing evidence that a Mediterranean-type moderate fat diet may also be useful in preventing CVD.

Additional information on nutrition and CVD is available at:
- Department of Health and Human Services
  Dietary Guidelines for Americans 2005
  http://www.healthierus.gov/dietaryguidelines

- National Center for Chronic Disease Prevention and Health Promotion
  Improving Nutrition and Increasing Physical Activity
  http://www.cdc,gov/nccdphp/bb_nutrition

9.6 CONTROL/NORMALIZE BLOOD PRESSURE

One of the key goals in preventing CVD is to control/normalize blood pressure through such means as diet, exercise, stress reduction and medication, if necessary.

The National Institute of Health DASH (Dietary Approaches to Stop Hypertension) diet has been found to be useful in controlling high blood pressure. This diet uses low-fat dairy foods and is rich in fruits and vegetables. It is low in total and saturated as well as trans fats, and reduces consumption of red meat, sweets, and sugar as well as "sugary" drinks. And the DASH diet also is rich in potassium, calcium, magnesium, fiber and protein.

Additional information regarding the DASH diet is available at:
- National Heart, Lung, and Blood Institute
  The DASH Eating Plan Puts Patients on the Road to Heart Health
  http://www.nhlbi.nih.gov/health/public/heart/hbp/dash
  The DASH Eating Plan
  http://www.nhlbi.nih.gov/health/public/heart/hbp/dash/new_dash.pdf

Weight loss and physical activity/exercise also help to lower/normalize blood pressure. In cases where diet, exercise and weight loss are not sufficient to "normalize" blood pressure, a number of prescription medications and strategies are now available. Such information is available at:

- American Academy of Family Physicians
  High Blood Pressure: Things You Can Do to Help Lower Yours
  http://www.familydoctor.org/092.xml
  Combination Antihypertensive Drugs: Recommendations for Use
  http://www.aafp.org/afp/20000515/3029/html

9.7 CONTROL/NORMALIZE BLOOD LIPIDS

As with blood pressure, eating a low to moderate fat, low cholesterol/saturated fat/trans fat diet, and engaging in a program of physical activity/exercise can improve blood lipid levels significantly. And, statin drugs represent a truly significant advance in the ability to "normalize" blood lipid levels and prevent CVD.

Additional information is available in section 8.4 and:

- American Academy of Family Practice
  Treatment of Cholesterol Abnormalities
  http://www.aafp.org/afp/20050315/1137.html

9.8 PREVENT/MANAGE DIABETES MELLITUS

The risk for CVD among persons with diabetes is 2 to 3 times higher than among persons without diabetes, and CVD accounts for 48 percent of all deaths among persons with diabetes.

Prevention via diet, exercise, control of body weight, and an active healthy lifestyle helps to reduce the risk of diabetes mellitus. Once established, satisfactory control of diabetes is essential in order to reduce the risk of CVD.

Additional information on diabetes and CVD is available at:

- American Diabetes Association
  Diabetes and Cardiovascular Disease
  http://www.diabetes.org
- Center for Disease Control and Prevention
  Cardiovascular Risk Factors and Related Preventive Health Practices Among Adults With and Without Diabetes
  http://www.cdc.gov/diabetes
- National Institute of Diabetes and Digestive and Kidney Disease
  The Link between Diabetes and Cardiovascular Disease
  http://www.niddk.nih.gov/diabetes/pubs/CVD_factsheet.pdf

9.9 PREVENT/MANAGE KIDNEY DISEASE

Chronic kidney disease (CKD) represents a significant risk for CVD. It needs to be prevented or it must be managed vigorously in order to minimize the risks.

Additional information on CVK and the relationship to CVD is available at:

- National Institute of Diabetes and Digestive and Kidney Diseases
  Kidney Disease Overview
  http://www.nkdep.nih.gov/healthprofessionals/ckdoverview.htm
  http://www.nkdep.nih.gov/patients.index.htm

9.10 STOP SMOKING/SECONDHAND SMOKE

Quit smoking and avoid secondhand smoke as much as possible in order to dramatically lower overall CVD risk. In the first year after quitting smoking, CVD risk drops sharply, and over time, risk generally returns to normal levels—like one who has never smoked or been exposed to chronic secondhand smoke.

Additional information is available at:
- American Academy of Family Physicians
  Smoking: Steps to Help You Break the Habit
  http://www.familydoctor.org/161.xml
- American Heart Association
  Smoking Cessation
  http://www.americanheart.org/presenter.jhtml?identifier=4731

9.11 REDUCE/COPE WITH STRESS

One needs to learn what stress is all about, how to handle the emotional problems of every day living, and cope with stress in life. Stress management is an integral part of any healthy lifestyle in order to minimize the effect of stress on the development of CVD.

In the final analysis, one of the best prescriptions for coping with stress is to adopt a healthy lifestyle. The principles and practices that may contribute to a less stressful healthy lifestyle, are summarized below:
- alcohol use should be sparing or not at all
- believe and have confidence in yourself
- choose a physician/healthcare facility prudently

- have an annual medical checkup
- control risk factors for disease
- take charge, control and responsibility for your life and health
- communicate effectively with others
- develop and maintain a rich and fulfilling spiritual life
- do good by others and your environment
- avoid intentional harm to yourself, others or anything
- minimize procrastination
- eat in healthy, nutritiously sound ways
- exercise regularly and maintain fitness
- follow good safety rules and avoid injuries
- follow a laudable purpose in life
- maintain good relationships
- make the world a better place
- moderate living/playing experiences and avoid excesses
- practice love, compassion, forgiveness, patience, understanding, meditation, mindfulness, prayer and self-control
- perform good body/oral and mental hygiene daily
- practice safe sex
- sleep regularly and restfully
- set and accomplish reasonable goals and objectives
- strive for emotional well being and control
- do not smoke/avoid secondhand smoke
- maintain normal weight

Living a healthy lifestyle and reducing and/or coping with stress increases in direct proportion to the successful incorporation of the above listed principles and practices into one's life.

Prayer also can play an important role not only in reducing stress but also in helping one cope with the stress in one's life. A good example of such a prayer is "The Serenity Prayer", presented in full text below.

God grant me the:

- Serenity to accept the things I cannot change, and
- Courage to change the things I can, and the
- Wisdom to know the difference
- Living one day at a time
- Enjoying one moment at a time
- Accepting hardship as the pathway to peace
- Taking, as He did, this sinful world as it is, not as I would have it
- Trusting that He will make all things right if I surrender to His will
- That I may be reasonably happy in this life, and supremely happy with Him forever in the next. Amen

Reinhold Neibuhr 1926

In dealing with stress and the emotional problems of everyday living, it also is important to remember the essence of the following from "The Way of All Flesh" which Dr. Karl Menninger has cited in his book, "The Human Kind", as one of the best definitions of the human mind—the true origin of all emotional stress.

"All our lives long, every day and every hour, we are engaged in the process of accommodating our changed and unchanged selves to changed and unchanged surrounding. Living, in fact is nothing else than this process of accommodation; when we fail in it a little we are stupid, when we fail flagrantly we are mad, when we suspend it temporarily we sleep, when we give up the attempt altogether we die. In quiet, uneventful lives the changes internal and external are so small that there is little or no strain in the process of fusion and accommodation; in other lives there is great strain, but there is also great fusing and accommodating power; in others great strain with little accommodating power. A life will be successful or not, according as the power of accommodation is equal to or unequal to the strain of fusing and adjusting internal and external changes."

Samuel Butler, "The Way of All Flesh" quoted in "The Human Mind" by Karl A. Menninger, Alfred A. Knoff, 1946

As pointed out by Sigmund Freud, in his book "Civilization and Its Discontents", civilization does breed its discontents and we all have to find effective ways to adapt/cope and effectively handle the emotional problems of every day life.

Additional information on stress is available at:

*   American Academy of Family Practice
    Stress: How to Cope Better With Life's Challenges
    http://www.familydoctor.org/167.html
    Stress: Who Has Time For It?
    http://www.familydoctor.org/xml
*   *Civilization and Its Discontents by Sigmund Freud*
    http://www.writing.upenn.edu/~afilreis/50s/freud-cir.html
*   National Institute of Mental Health
    Depression Can Break Your Heart
    http://www.nimh.nih.gov/heartbreak.fm

Depression and Heart Disease

http://www.nimh.nih.gov/publicat/deheart.cfm

- Mind Body Medical Institute

  Stress Management/Mindfulness

  http://www.mbmi.org

CHAPTER 10

▼

AUTHOR'S LIST: CVD WEB RESOURCES/WEBSITES

1. Agency for Healthcare Research and Quality
    http://www.ahrq.gov
2. American Academy of Family Physicians
    http://www.aafp.org
    http://familydoctor.org
3. American Academy of Periodontology
    http://www.perio.org
4. American College of Cardiology
    http://www.acc.org
5. American College of Physicians
    http://www.acponline.org
6. American College of Preventive Medicine
    http://www.acpm.org
7. American Dental Association
    http://www.ada.org
8. American Diabetes Association
    http://www.diabetes.org

9. American Heart Association
   http://www.americanheart.org
10. American Medical Association
    http://www.ama-assn.org
11. Centers for Disease Control and Prevention
    http://www.cdc.gov
12. Cleveland Clinic Heart Center
    http://www.clevelandclinic.org/heartcenter
13. FDA Heart Health Online
    http://www.fda.gov/hearthealth/riskfactors/riskfactors.html
    http://www.fda.gov/fdac/features/2003/603_heart.html
14. Food and Drug Administration
    http://www.fda.gov
15. Harvard Medical School/Consumer Health Information
    http://www.intelihealth.com
16. Harvard School of Public Health
    http://www.hsph.harvard.edu
17. Healthfinder
    http://www.healthfinder.gov
18. Healthy People 2010
    http://www.healthypeople.gov/BeHealthy
19. Johns Hopkins Bloomberg School of Public Health
    http://www.jhsph.edu
20. Just Move
    http://www.justmove.org
21. Lab Tests Online
    http://www.labtestsonline.net

22. Medlineplus
    http://www.medlineplus.gov
23. Mind/Body Medical Institute
    http://www.mbmi.org
24. National Center for Chronic Disease Prevention and Health Promotion
    http://www.cdc.nccdphp/bb_heartdisease/index.htm
25. National Cholesterol Education Program
    http://www.nhlbi.nih.gov/about/ncep/index.htm
26. National Heart, Lung and Blood Institute
    http://www.nhlbi.nih.gov
27. National Institute of Diabetes and Digestive and Kidney Disease
    http://www.niddk.nih.gov
28. National Institute of Health/Health Information
    http://www.health.nih.gov
29. National Institute of Mental Health
    http://www.nimh.nih.gov
30. National Institute of Neurological Disorders and Stroke
    http://www.ninds.gov
    http://www.ninds.nih.gov/disorders/stroke/preventing_stroke_pr.htm
31. National Stroke Association
    http://stroke.org
32. National Women's Health Information Center
    http://www.4women.gov/faq/heartdis.htm
33. Nutrition Institute of America
    http://www.nutritioninstituteofamerica.org
34. Penn State Heart and Vascular Institute
    http://www.hmc.psu.edu/heartandvascular

35. Texas Heart Institute
   http://www.texasheartinstitute.org/riskfact.html

36. UCLA School of Medicine
   http://www.ucla.edu

37. UCLA Stroke Center
   http://www.stroke.mednet.ucla.edu/links.html

38. World Health Organization
   http://www.who.int

CHAPTER 11

▼

SEARCHING THE WEB

Although search engines such as Google may provide reasonably complete searches of the Web, one is left with the very difficult and time consuming task of reviewing many thousands or more Web pages/reports provided after a search in order to determine which contain reasonably trustworthy, current, comprehensive and useful information. Unfortunately, this usually is well beyond the capability of all but a few readers to accomplish satisfactorily in a reasonable period of time.

In order to simplify matters in this regard, the author has carefully selected, personally reviewed, and assembled the Author's List: CVD Resources/ Websites in Chapter 10 that are considered to be most useful overall for CVD information pertaining to the scope of material presented in this book, and has listed them alphabetically for ease of reference. Each of these Web resources/websites provides a Search site and links that may be used to obtain additional information.

This Author's List provides reasonably reliable, up-to-date CVD information assembled by professional organizations, medical schools, or official US government resources.

In instituting any search for CVD information using the Author's List, it is important to remember that the Web is growing rapidly, and is in a constant state of flux, updating and reorganization. Web resources provided may change/modify their name and/or website address, format, content and categorization/display of information, as well as delete or change Web pages/reports.

If for any reason, the website chosen for a report doesn't work, search the Web resource name itself for the desired information. Should a problem still persist, try another search engine to access the Web resource and/or website in question.

Web resources use different methods to search the Web to compile their databases. Each Web resource organizes/assembles information differently, some more complete, current, and easier to use than others. Thus, different Web resources/websites likely will provide information that may differ significantly and need to be reconciled. And, Web pages/reports/information may be changed or removed or temporarily become unavailable on any given Web resource/website for a number of reasons.

In general, the CVD information obtained via the Author's List may be regarded as reasonably reliable and useful in most instances/respects but not necessarily all. Unlike medical/scientific articles published in peer review journals, here is no guarantee that CVD information obtained from any single Web resource/website in the Author's List may necessarily be relied upon as the "gospel truth". Therefore, information from a minimum of at least two to three other Web resources/websites need to be compared and reconciled, when different. Also, in the amazing world of the Web, a second or even a third opinion is considered to be worthwhile. Even in the case of scientific, evidence-based information from well-controlled trials, there may be problems in terms of what the data collected/results may mean. Clinical trial evidence necessarily is subject to interpretation and application, both subjective processes. Everyone is biased to some degree in one way or another in obtaining, analyzing, interpreting and applying information, evidence based or not. Words, phrases, statistics, conclusions, etc. mean different things to different people at different times and places, depending on "where one is coming from" so to speak. For example, even in the case of the Constitution of the United States of America, written by "great minds"—individuals, lawyers, judges, senators and representatives, and even the Supreme Court members still continue to debate, argue, disagree about and usually have great difficulty interpreting and applying the so-called "original intent" of the founding fathers/authors of this great document.

Nevertheless, one may entertain a certain degree of confidence that the CVD information obtained via the Web resources/websites in this book may help one become better informed in order to help prevent CVD and live a healthier, happier, longer, and more productive/enjoyable life.

▼

CHAPTER 12

ABOUT THE AUTHOR

Eugene A. DeFelice is an internationally recognized author, educator, and retired Distinguished Clinical Professor Medicine, Robert Wood Johnson Medical School, 1977–2003. He is listed in the prestigious Marquis' Who's Who in Medicine and Healthcare, Who's Who in America, and Who's Who in the World. Dr. DeFelice is a Fellow of the Academy of Psychosomatic Medicine, and the American Geriatrics Society and author of over 65 medical/scientific articles and 11 books on medicine, nutrition, and health and Web health resources. Books published include:

1. Prevention of Cardiovascular Disease, iUniverse Inc., 2005

2. Web Health Information Resources, Second Edition, iUniverse Inc., 2004

3. Nutrition and Health, iUniverse Inc., 2003

4. Overweight, Obesity and Health, iUniverse Inc., 2002

5. Breast Cancer, iUniverse Inc., 2002

6. Web Health Information Resource Guide, iUniverse Inc., 2001

7. Angiotension Converting Enzyme Inhibitor, Alan R. Liss, 1987

8. Pharmacological Treatment of Cardiovascular Disease, Elsevier, 1986

9. Beta Blockers in the Treatment of Cardiovascular Disease, Raven Press, 1984

10. Health and Obesity, Raven Press, 1983
11. Prostaglandins, Platelets, Lipids: New Developments in Atherosclerosis, Elsevier, 1981

978-0-595-36884-6
0-595-36884-0